Nursing care

The Burns Unit:

The Complete Guide

ALEXANDRE CAREWELL

Table of contents

4

« Every patient in the burns unit is a phoenix, rising from the ashes with a strength and determination that only those who have been through the fire can understand. »

Chapter 1:
INTRODUCTION TO THE BURN UNIT

History and
development treatment of burns

The treatment of burns through the ages reflects both humanity's journey in understanding the human body and our ingenuity in healing and restoring it. This age-old quest for healing is as old as humanity itself. Each era, each culture, has had its own way of perceiving and treating burns, and this history is fascinating.

In ancient times, long before we understood the science behind infections or the importance of infertility, treatments were based on natural remedies and traditions. The Egyptians, for example, used ointments made from honey, resin and other medicinal plants to treat burns. In addition to their curative properties, these substances were believed to ward off evil spirits. Hippocrates, the father of medicine, recommended the use of ointments to protect and moisturise burnt skin.

As civilisations progressed, surgery began to play a role in the treatment of serious burns. However, it was only in modern times, with the advent of medical science, that significant advances were made. The understanding of the importance of sterility, for example, radically changed the approach to treatment.

During the world wars of the 20th century, faced with an unprecedented number of burns caused by explosions and fires, the need to improve treatment techniques became imperative. It was during this period that the first skin bank was created, and the first skin grafts were performed. Research also made huge strides in understanding the physiology of burns, leading to better resuscitation and care techniques.

In recent decades, technology has opened up new horizons. Intelligent dressings capable of releasing drugs over an extended period, stem cells to regenerate skin, and even 3D printers to create skin grafts - all innovations that were unimaginable a century ago.

This journey through time, from ancient remedies based on tradition to modern solutions based on science, illustrates not only our evolution as a medical society, but also our unwavering commitment to healing, relieving pain and restoring hope.

The crucial importance
of the burns unit

There are certain departments in the medical world whose role is so specific and delicate that they become almost sacred in their mission. The burns unit is one of these bastions of hope and healing, where every operation is a race against time, a delicate dance between science, art and compassion.

Burns, particularly severe ones, can cause irreversible damage not only to the skin, but also to the underlying tissues, muscles, tendons and even bones. This goes far beyond mere physical pain. The psychological, emotional and social implications of living with a severe burn are profound. Disfigurement, loss of mobility, emotional scars - all these consequences require a holistic approach to treatment and rehabilitation.

That's where the burns unit comes in. It's not just a place where physical injuries are treated. It's a sanctuary where a multidisciplinary team - surgeons, nurses, psychologists, occupational therapists and others - come together to offer patients not only a chance of survival, but also of regaining a quality of life.

In this department, every detail counts. Precise fluid management to avoid shock; the prevention of infections, which can be fatal in an environment where the skin's first line of defence is compromised; skin grafting to restore the protective barrier; physiotherapy to regain mobility; and psychological intervention to help patients rebuild their self-esteem and face the world with their scars - these are all part of the day-to-day life of the burns unit.

But beyond science and technology, this service is a testament to the resilience of the human spirit. Every patient who comes in with injuries is a reminder of our vulnerability, but every patient who emerges healed is a testament to our ability to overcome, adapt and be reborn.

The importance of the burns service is measured not just in terms of lives saved, but also in terms of lives transformed, hopes restored and dreams renewed. It is a beacon of humanity within the medical world, illustrating what we can achieve when science, compassion and determination meet.

Mission and vision of the nurse in this department

At the heart of the burns unit, the nurse plays a central role, acting not only as guardian of the patient's health, but also as guide, support and ally in the healing process. The mission and vision of the nurse in this department reflect a deep commitment to the holistic wellbeing of the patient.

Mission:

The nurse's primary mission in the burns unit is to provide high-quality medical care, focusing on patient safety and comfort. They provide continuous monitoring, administer prescribed treatments, prevent potential complications and intervene quickly if there is any change in the patient's state of health. The nurse is also an essential communicator, acting as a link between the patient, the family and the medical team, ensuring optimum coordination of care.

However, the nurse's mission goes beyond medical interventions. Thanks to their constant proximity to the patient, nurses are often the first to recognise and respond to emotional and psychological needs. In an environment where patients are confronted with intense pain, fear and uncertainty, the nurse offers an attentive ear, a reassuring hand and a compassionate heart.

Vision :

The nurse's vision extends beyond the hospital room. It envisions a world where every patient, despite hardship and trauma, can return to a life full of dignity, functionality and joy. To achieve this vision, nurses constantly strive to improve their skills, keep abreast of the latest advances in burn care, and promote a culture of excellence and empathy within the care team.

This vision also encompasses the importance of education and prevention. The nurse, as educator, plays a crucial role in teaching patients and their families about home care, rehabilitation and the prevention of future injuries.

At the heart of this mission and vision is an unwavering commitment to humanity. For the burns nurse, every day is an opportunity to combine science with compassion, skill with care, with the ultimate goal of restoring not only the patient's physical health, but also their mind and soul.

Chapter 2:
BASIC UNDERSTANDING OF BURNS

Classification of burns

• First-degree burns

The skin is our first line of defence against external aggression, acting as both a physical barrier and a sensitive sensor. Burns are injuries that can partially or totally affect these functions, depending on their severity. Of the various classifications of burns, first-degree burns are the most superficial, but this does not mean that they should be neglected or taken lightly.

Features :
First-degree burns only affect the outermost layer of the skin, the epidermis. They are generally characterised by :
- Redness of the skin (erythema).
- Mild to moderate pain, often described as a burning or tingling sensation.
- Dry, blister-free skin.
- Increased sensitivity in the affected area.

The most common cause of this type of burn is brief exposure to a heat source, such as sunburn, contact with hot water or a brief encounter with a flame or heated surface.

Treatment :
- **Immediate cooling:** Following a first-degree burn, it is essential to cool the affected area. This can be done by gently running the burned area under cold water for several minutes.

- **Avoid direct application of ice:** Although cooling is crucial, direct application of ice can cause further damage to the skin.
- **Moisturising and care:** Applying a moisturising lotion or aloe vera gel can help relieve pain and prevent the skin from peeling.
- **Avoid exposure:** It is advisable to protect the burned area from the sun and other sources of heat while it heals.

Course and prognosis :
First-degree burns are generally benign and heal on their own within a few days. The skin may peel during the healing process, but this should not be a cause for concern. However, if the burn is extensive, particularly in the case of sunburn over a large part of the body, it is essential to consult a health professional. In addition, any burn on the face, hands, feet or genitals, even if it seems superficial, should be assessed by a professional.

Although first-degree burns are the least serious in the classification of burns, appropriate management and attention to the signs of complications ensure rapid recovery with no after-effects.

• Second-degree burns
While it is true that all burns lead to a disruption in the integrity of the skin, second-degree burns, by their very nature, present a particular challenge. They affect not only the epidermis, but also part or all of the dermis, the layer of skin just below it. Second-degree burns are often more painful and present a higher risk of complications than first-degree burns.

Features :
Second-degree burns are distinguished by :

- The appearance of blisters on the skin.
- Intense redness.
- Marked pain.
- Skin that may appear shiny or damp due to the fluid contained in the blisters.
- Increased sensitivity.

Common causes:
The causes of these burns can vary: prolonged contact with a flame, hot water or liquids, electrical contact, chemical reactions or prolonged exposure to the sun.

Treatment :
- **Cooling:** As with first-degree burns, cooling the affected area by running it under cold water for at least 10 minutes is a crucial step.
- **Protecting the burn:** Once the burn has cooled, it is essential to protect it to prevent infection. This can be done using sterile plastic film or a non-adhesive dressing.
- **Do not pierce blisters:** Although they can be uncomfortable, blisters play a protective role. Their liquid is sterile and acts as a cushion against rubbing and external aggression.
- **Painkillers:** Second-degree burns can be very painful, and taking painkillers can help relieve the pain.
- **Moisturising:** After a few days, once healing has begun, regular moisturising of the area can help prevent flaking and itching.

Course and prognosis :
Second-degree burns require careful monitoring to detect any complications, particularly infections. Healing can take from a few days to a few weeks, depending on the depth of the burn. Deep second-degree burns can leave scars,

which is why it is important to consult a professional to assess the severity of the burn.

Although second-degree burns are more serious than first-degree burns, appropriate treatment, regular follow-up and prevention of complications can help ensure optimal healing.

• **Third-degree burns**

Third-degree burns are one of the most severe injuries the skin can sustain. They penetrate the entire thickness of the skin, destroying not only the epidermis and dermis, but also often reaching underlying tissues such as fat, tendons and sometimes even bone.

Features :
Unlike less severe burns, the characteristics of third-degree burns include :
Skin that may appear whitish, charred or dark.
A leathery or waxy texture.
A lack of sensitivity in the affected area due to the destruction of nerve endings.
No blisters.

Common causes:
Third-degree burns are generally caused by prolonged contact with a flame, corrosive chemicals, an electric current or extremely hot liquids.

Treatment :
Medical emergency: Third-degree burns require immediate medical attention. The first step is to call emergency or go to the nearest burns unit.

Do not remove stuck-on clothing: If clothing has melted or stuck to the burn, do not attempt to remove it.

Avoid hydration: Unlike less serious burns, it is not recommended to cool a third-degree burn with water, as this can aggravate the injury or cause shock.

Protection from infection: Because of the severity of the burn, it is crucial to protect it from contaminants until medical intervention can take place.

Course and prognosis :
The treatment of third-degree burns is often complex. It generally requires hospitalisation, surgical interventions such as skin grafts and a long period of rehabilitation. The risk of infection is very high, and is one of the main concerns in treatment.

Scarring is almost always a consequence of these burns, and physiotherapy may be required to maintain mobility in the affected area. In addition, because of the psychological impact of such injuries, the patient may benefit from psychological support or therapy.

Third-degree burns, although severe and often traumatic, are not insurmountable. With medical advances, the support of care teams and the resilience of the patient, recovery, albeit long, is possible.

• **Fourth-degree burns**

Fourth-degree burns are the most serious and deepest of all burn classifications. They not only affect all layers of the skin, but also extend to underlying structures such as muscles, tendons and sometimes even bones.

Features :
The seriousness of fourth-degree burns is evident from the following symptoms:

Charred skin, which may be black or coal-like.
Hard or crunchy texture of the affected area.

- Total lack of sensitivity due to complete destruction of the nerves.
- In some cases, the bone may be visible.

Common causes:
These burns can be caused by electrocution, prolonged exposure to flames or highly corrosive chemicals, and sometimes even extremely cold temperatures (deep frostbite).

Treatment :

Urgent medical intervention : In the event of a fourth-degree burn, emergency medical intervention is absolutely crucial. The individual must be taken immediately to a centre specialising in the treatment of burns.

Avoid touching or trying to treat the burn: Given the severity of the lesion, it's best to avoid any unprofessional intervention.

Avoid water: As with third-degree burns, do not attempt to cool the burn with water.

Cover the area: If possible, cover the burn with a sterile cloth or clean bandage to protect it while waiting for medical attention.

Course and prognosis :
Fourth-degree burns are complex injuries requiring multiple surgical interventions, including amputations or bone grafts. Even with appropriate medical intervention, the after-effects can be permanent, such as loss of function of a body part, deep scars or deformities.

Treatment is not limited to the acute phase. Patients may require lengthy rehabilitation, intensive physiotherapy and psychological support to overcome the trauma of the injury.

When faced with a burn of this magnitude, the emphasis is not only on physical healing, but also on psychological and social support to help patients reintegrate into society and regain a sense of normality in their lives. Resilience, family support and a dedicated medical team are essential to navigating the long road to recovery.

Common causes
serious burns

Serious burns can occur for a variety of reasons, but some causes are more common than others. Understanding these causes is essential not only for treatment, but also for prevention.

Flames and fire :

Domestic accidents: These can result from kitchen fires, spilled candles or careless handling of combustibles.

Industrial accidents: Explosions or uncontrolled fires on industrial sites can cause serious burns to workers.

Vehicles: Accidents involving cars or other vehicles can sometimes cause fires, exposing victims to open flames.

Hot liquids (scalding) :

Often linked to domestic accidents such as spilling boiling water, soups or cooking oil.

In industrial environments, leaks of pressurised liquids or vapours can also cause burns.

Chemical products :

Acids and bases: Mainly found in laboratories, industrial sites and even some household products.

Reagents: Some chemicals can react violently when in contact with other substances or when exposed to air or water.

Toxic gases: Inhaling chemical gases can burn the internal respiratory tract.

Electrocution :

Domestic accidents: Caused by faulty electrical installations or unsafe handling of electrical appliances.

Industrial accidents: Workers may come into contact with high-voltage lines or live equipment.

Radiation :

Prolonged   exposure to the sun: This can cause burns, particularly in very sunny environments or when exposed without adequate protection.

Ionising radiation: In very specific contexts, such as industrial radiography or certain medical procedures, unprotected exposure can cause burns.

Contact with extremely hot   surfaces:

This could include stoves, irons, engine exhaust pipes or any other heated surface.

Extreme   cold (frostbite) :

Although not always classified as 'burns' in the traditional sense, frostbite is technically a burn caused by the cold. They can occur from prolonged exposure to freezing temperatures without adequate protection.

Knowledge of the common causes of serious burns is crucial for nurses, as it enables rapid assessment of the situation, appropriate treatment and prevention of possible complications. But beyond treatment, raising awareness of these causes is also a powerful tool for preventing and reducing the number of burn-related accidents.

Pathophysiology of burns

Burn pathophysiology describes the biological changes and mechanisms that occur at cellular and systemic level after a burn injury. This knowledge is fundamental to understanding the severity of burns, as well as establishing an effective treatment plan.

Immediate reaction (local inflammatory response):

Initial vasoconstriction: Immediately after the burn, the blood vessels in the affected area temporarily contract.

Vasodilatation: Rapidly followed by dilation of the blood vessels, leading to redness, heat and oedema.

Release of inflammatory mediators: Damaged cells release substances such as histamines, cytokines and prostaglandins, which amplify the inflammatory response.

Cellular damage :

Protein denaturation: Heat causes cell proteins to coagulate, leading to cell death.

Membrane disintegration: The cell membrane may be compromised, causing the release of enzymes and other intracellular components into the surrounding tissue.

Burn zones (according to Jackson's concentric zone theory) :

Coagulation zone: Located in the centre of the burn, this is the most damaged area where the cells have died.

Zone of ischaemia (or stasis): The cells here are damaged but not dead. With appropriate treatment, they can survive.

Zone of hyperaemia: This is the peripheral zone where the cells have been affected by the burn, but are likely to recover without intervention.

Systemic response :

Systemic inflammatory response: In extensive burns, inflammation is not limited to the burned area. Inflammatory mediators are released into the circulation, which can lead to an inflammatory response throughout the body.

Compromised immune response: Burns can affect the body's ability to fight infection, increasing the risk of secondary infections.

Fluid imbalance: Severe burns can lead to significant fluid loss, requiring rehydration.

Long-term complications :

Healing: The healing of burns can lead to the formation of hypertrophic or keloid scars.

Functional restrictions: Deep burns can affect tendons, muscles and joints, limiting mobility.

Dyspigmentation: Burned areas may heal with altered pigmentation, either being darker or lighter than the surrounding skin.

Understanding the pathophysiology of burns is essential for nurses and other healthcare professionals. It helps them to anticipate patient needs, monitor potential complications and establish effective care strategies to improve outcomes.

Chapter 3:
THE ROLE OF THE NURSE: FIRST CONTACT AND INITIAL ASSESSMENT

Welcoming the patient: First look and psychological support

Welcoming a patient with burns is a crucial moment in their care. The first contact with the nursing staff can have a considerable influence on the patient's perception of their situation and their emotional state. In this context, the role of the nurse is crucial.

Initial assessment :

Safety: The first step is to ensure that the patient is safe and that the cause of the burn has been eliminated.

Medical assessment: First and foremost, the nurse must quickly assess the severity of the burn, the airways, breathing and circulation, and the degree of pain.

Empathetic communication :

Make eye contact: Reassuring eye contact can help build trust.

Active listening: Nurses must listen carefully to patients, allowing them to express their concerns and pain.

Body language: An open, attentive posture shows patients that they are being cared for and listened to.

Psychological support :

Reassurance: Informing the patient that everything is being done to look after him or her. Clarity about the steps ahead can reduce anxiety.

Validation: Acknowledging the patient's pain and distress without minimising their feelings.

Orientation: Explaining to the patient where they are, what is going to happen next and who is there to support them.

Assessment of mental well-being :

Rapid screening: Quickly identify signs of acute emotional or psychological distress, such as agitation, confusion or apathy.

Team support: Involve psychologists or psychiatrists as soon as necessary to assess and intervene in cases of emotional trauma.

Family and friends :

Communication: Informing the family of the patient's condition and the next steps.

Support: Recognising and responding to the emotional distress of loved ones, who may also need support.

Long-term monitoring :

Therapy: Severe burns can lead to post-burn trauma. Therapy can help manage stress, depression and other emotional reactions.

Support groups: Support groups can provide a platform for burn victims to share their experiences and challenges.

Welcoming a burn victim is much more than a simple medical assessment. It is the start of a relationship of trust, emotional support and an affirmation that the patient is in an environment where they will be cared for, respected and supported throughout their convalescence.

Assessment of severity: Body surface area and depth

Determining the severity of a burn is crucial for guiding therapeutic management and anticipating potential complications. Two essential aspects must be taken into account: the extent of the burn, often expressed as a percentage of the total body surface area (TSA) burnt, and the depth of the burn.

Assessment of the body surface area affected :

Rule of 9: A commonly used technique for rapidly estimating burned TSS in adults. The body surface is divided into multiple regions, each representing approximately 9% (or a multiple of 9%) of the total TSS.

Head and neck: 9%.
Each arm: 9
Thorax: 18
Back: 18
Each leg: 18
Perineal area: 1

Palmar Method: Uses the surface area of the patient's palm (not including the fingers) as representing approximately 1% of the TBS.

Paediatrics: Proportions differ in children. As a result, specific maps (such as the Lund and Browder diagram) are used to estimate TSC burnt in children.

Assessing the depth of the burn :

First-degree burn :
Only affects the epidermis.
Redness, pain, slight swelling.
Heals in a few days without scarring.
Second-degree burn :

27

Affects the epidermis and part or all of the dermis.

Can be superficial (red, painful, blistering) or deep (whitish or mottled, less painful).

Requires care to prevent infection and reduce scarring.

Third-degree burn :

Complete destruction of the epidermis and dermis.

White, brown or blackish appearance.

Insensitive to touch. Often requires skin grafting.

Fourth degree burn :

Penetrates subcutaneous structures such as muscles, tendons and even bones.

Charred appearance.

Surgery and long-term rehabilitation are often necessary.

Consideration of aggravating factors:

Location: Burns to the face, hands, feet, joints or genital area may require special attention.

Age: Children and the elderly may have a more severe reaction and a slower recovery.

Other trauma: Patients with burns associated with other trauma, such as fractures, may have increased complications.

Underlying medical conditions: Conditions such as diabetes or cardiovascular disease can influence the severity of the burn and the response to treatment.

The ability to accurately assess the extent and depth of a burn is essential for defining an optimal treatment plan. It enables fluid requirements to be adjusted, surgical needs to be anticipated and nursing care to be guided throughout recovery.

Drawing up an initial care plan

Drawing up an initial care plan for a burn patient is a crucial step that determines not only immediate interventions, but also medium- and long-term care. This plan is drawn up on the basis of the previous assessment of the patient's severity and specific needs.

Initial stabilisation :

ABC (Airway, Breathing, Circulation): Before any other intervention, it is crucial to ensure airway patency, check breathing and assess circulation.

Pain treatment: Administer analgesics according to the severity of the pain.

Initial assessment: Carry out an assessment of vital functions, blood sugar levels and other parameters, depending on the patient's clinical condition.

Burn assessment and care :

Cleaning: Remove clothing and debris and gently clean the burnt area.

Application of an antibiotic ointment: To prevent infection and moisturise the skin.

Dressing: Use sterile dressings appropriate to the severity and location of the burn.

Rehydration :

Calculating fluid requirements: Based on the TSC burnt, the patient's age and weight.

Choice of solute: Electrolyte solutions such as lactated Ringer's are commonly used.

Monitoring: Monitor closely for signs of overhydration or dehydration.

Infection prevention :

Aseptic techniques: Handle burns with sterile gloves and keep the environment clean.

Monitoring: Watch for signs of infection, such as increased pain, redness, pus or fever.

Antibiotics: To be considered in the event of signs of infection or according to the establishment's protocol.

Nutrition :

Needs assessment: Burn patients often have increased calorie requirements.

Diet: Encourage a diet rich in proteins and calories.

Emotional and psychological   support :

Assessment: Identifying signs of distress or trauma.

Guidance: Involve psychologists or social workers depending on the patient's needs.

Communication :

With the team: Ensuring that information is properly passed on between the various care teams.

With the patient and family: Keeping the patient and family informed of interventions, progress and prospects.

Short-term   planning :

Regular assessments: Plan regular assessments of the burn, pain, nutrition, etc.

Physiotherapy: Start as soon as possible to prevent retractions and promote mobility.

Drawing up an initial care plan is a dynamic process that requires constant reassessment and adjustment. The active involvement of the nurse, with his or her clinical skills and empathy, is fundamental to ensuring optimal care for the burn patient.

Chapter 4:
SPECIFIC TECHNIQUES AND CARE

Disinfecting and cleaning the burn

Disinfection and cleaning of burns are fundamental steps in preventing infectious complications, promoting healing and reducing the risk of unwanted scarring. These procedures require a great deal of expertise, as they must be carried out delicately to avoid aggravating existing tissue damage.

Initial assessment :

Visual inspection: Check for debris, clothing, soot or other contaminants.

Sensitivity assessment: Understanding the patient's pain level to adapt analgesia.

Preparing the patient :

Analgesia: Analgesics should be administered prior to the start of cleaning to ensure patient comfort. Analgesia may be systemic, topical or a combination of both.

Explanation: Tell the patient what you are going to do to reduce anxiety.

Cleaning technique :

Using lukewarm water: The water should be at a comfortable temperature to avoid any additional thermal shock.

Gentle cleaning: Use a sterile saline solution or a mild cleanser to gently remove any debris or soot. Use gentle movements to avoid aggravating the lesion.

Avoid rubbing: Do not rub the burn. This could cause further damage.

Disinfection :

> **Antiseptic agents:** Solutions such as povidone-iodine or chlorhexidine can be used. However, some antiseptics can delay healing, so it is essential to follow the establishment's recommendations.

> **Antibiotic ointments:** Can be applied after cleaning to prevent infection.

Rinsing :

> After cleaning and disinfection, rinse the burn thoroughly with sterile water or saline solution to remove any residue.

Drying :

> **Dab gently:** Use a soft cloth or sterile gauze to dry the burn. Avoid rubbing.

> **Preparation for dressing:** Make sure the area is dry before applying the dressing to avoid maceration.

Monitoring :

> **Signs of infection:** After cleaning, monitor the area regularly for signs of infection such as increasing redness, pus, foul odour or fever in the patient.

Disinfecting and cleaning burns are essential steps that require meticulousness and delicacy. The nurse's skill in this procedure is vital to ensure optimal healing and reduce potential complications.

Debridement:
Importance and methods

Debridement is an essential medical process in the management of burns, as it removes necrotic (dead) and contaminated tissue from the burn surface. Removing this tissue facilitates healing, reduces the risk of infection and improves the aesthetic appearance of the final scar. This is a delicate stage that requires expertise and precision.

The importance of debridement :

Infection prevention : Necrotic tissue can become a breeding ground for bacteria.

Facilitates healing: By removing non-viable tissue, debridement encourages the growth of new, healthy tissue.

Reduced scarring: Proper debridement can minimise the formation of unsightly or contracted scars.

Debridement methods :

Surgical debridement :

This is the quickest and most common method.

It involves the use of surgical instruments to mechanically remove necrotic tissue.

This procedure may require a local or general anaesthetic.

Enzymatic debridement :

This method uses topical enzymes to dissolve necrotic tissue.

It is less invasive than surgical debridement and is often used for smaller burns or as a complement to surgery.

Autolytic debridement :

This is a natural method that uses the patient's own body enzymes.

Occlusive or hydrogel dressings are used to maintain a moist environment, encouraging autolysis of necrotic tissue.

It is a slower process, but less painful and invasive.

Mechanical debridement :

This may involve using a damp gauze that is left to dry over the burn, then removing it, taking the necrotic tissue with it as it is removed.

Although this method is simpler, it can be painful and can also remove healthy tissue.

Biological debridement :

Uses sterilised maggots from certain species of flies to break down and consume necrotic tissue without harming living tissue.

It is an effective method, but it may not be well accepted by all patients due to its nature.

Care after debridement :

Dressings: Depending on the debridement method, specific dressings will be required to protect the area, promote healing and prevent infection.

Pain control: Debridement can be painful. It is essential to monitor and manage the patient's pain proactively.

Monitoring for signs of infection: Despite debridement, the risk of infection remains. It is therefore crucial to observe the treated area carefully.

Debridement, when carried out correctly and at the right time, plays a crucial role in the treatment of burns. The choice of method will depend on the severity of the burn, its location and the patient's preferences and needs. The nurse's skill in this area is essential to ensure the best possible care and promote optimal healing.

Pain management:
Medicines and non-medicinal methods

Pain management is central to the care of patients with severe burns. It requires a holistic approach, combining pharmacological and non-pharmacological interventions to provide optimal relief and promote healing.

Pain management drugs :
Non-opioid analgesics :
Paracetamol (Acetaminophen): This is often used for mild to moderate pain.

NSAIDs (such as ibuprofen): These can reduce pain and inflammation. However, they should be used with caution in certain patients because of possible side effects.
Opiates :
Morphine, Fentanyl, Oxycodone: These drugs are used for moderate to severe pain. They must be administered under close supervision due to their side effects and the risk of dependence.
Adjuvant analgesics :
Certain anticonvulsants and antidepressants can be used to complement pain management, particularly neuropathic pain.
Local anaesthetics :
Lidocaine, bupivacaine: These medicines can be used in topical or injectable form to numb a specific area.
Non-medicinal methods :
Physical therapies :
Hydrotherapy: Warm water can help clean wounds while providing pain relief.

Physiotherapy: Controlled movement can prevent contractures and help manage pain.

Relaxation and distraction techniques :

Meditation and deep breathing: These techniques can help relax the body and mind, reducing the perception of pain.

Music therapy: Listening to music can be an excellent distraction and can also have a calming effect.

Art therapy: Drawing, painting or modelling with clay can help patients express their feelings while distracting them from the pain.

Psychological interventions :

Cognitive-behavioural therapy: This approach can help patients to develop strategies for managing their pain.

Hypnotherapy: Some patients find relief through hypnosis.

Complementary therapies :

Acupuncture and acupressure: These techniques can help relieve pain by stimulating certain points on the body.

Massage: This can relax muscles and improve circulation, helping to reduce pain.

Managing pain in burn patients is a complex task that requires a personalised approach. A combination of medication and non-medication methods is often the key to ensuring patient comfort, promoting healing and preventing the long-term complications associated with poorly managed pain.

Dressing techniques and skin grafts

When it comes to treating burns, dressings and skin grafts are fundamental elements. The choice of dressing or grafting technique depends on the severity of the burn, its location and the patient's general condition.

Dressing techniques :

Wet-dry dressings: This method involves applying a wet compress to the burn, which is then covered with a dry bandage. This allows the wound to be cleaned when the dressing is changed.

Hydrocolloid dressings: Composed of a gel-forming matrix, they maintain a moist environment that promotes healing while protecting against infection.

Hydrogel dressings: These dressings are mainly composed of water and provide essential moisture to the wound, facilitating healing and autolytic debridement.

Alginate dressings: Made from brown seaweed, they are particularly absorbent and suitable for exudative wounds.

Silver dressings : Silver is an antimicrobial agent. These dressings are used to prevent or treat infections in burn wounds.

Polyurethane films: These are semi-permeable dressings that allow gas exchange while retaining moisture, suitable for superficial burns.

Skin grafts :

Autologous transplants :

Thin epidermal grafts: Removal of a thin layer of the patient's own epidermis. They are often used for large burned areas.

Full-thickness grafts: These include the epidermis and part of the dermis. They offer a better aesthetic and functional result, but the donor area also requires a graft or suture.

Allografts: Tissues taken from a human donor, often used as a temporary solution while waiting for an autologous transplant.

Xenografts: Tissues taken from animals, usually pigs. They are used as a temporary solution because of the risk of rejection.

Synthetic grafts :

Integra: A skin substitute with a collagen layer for the dermis and a silicone membrane for the temporary epidermis.

Dermagraft: Made from human fibroblasts, it is used to help regenerate the dermis.

Keratinocyte cultures: For patients with large burned areas, skin cells can be cultured in the laboratory and then applied to the wound.

Mastery of dressing techniques and skin grafts is essential to ensure optimal healing for burn patients. Every patient is unique, so it is crucial to regularly assess and review treatment options to adapt to the changing needs of the wound and the patient. Multidisciplinary collaboration between nurses, surgeons and other healthcare professionals is essential to provide the best possible care.

Chapter 5:
NUTRITIONAL CHALLENGES AND METABOLIC

Understanding post-burn catabolism

Post-burn catabolism refers to the acceleration of metabolism that occurs after a severe burn. It is a complex physiological response involving many body systems, and understanding it is crucial to the optimal management of burn patients.

The basics of catabolism :
Catabolism is the process of breaking down complex molecules into simpler ones in the body, releasing energy. In the post-burn context, this process is accelerated, leading to increased muscle breakdown and other systemic effects.

Triggers of post-burn catabolism :
Inflammation: A burn provokes an intense inflammatory response that releases cytokines and other pro-inflammatory mediators. These substances stimulate catabolism.

Stress: Burns are a serious form of trauma for the body, triggering the release of stress hormones such as cortisol, which also promote catabolism.

Forced fasting: Discomfort and pain can reduce the patient's food intake, contributing to catabolism.

Consequences of post-burn catabolism :

Muscle loss: Increased protein breakdown leads to significant muscle loss, affecting the patient's strength and mobility.

Organ atrophy: Like muscles, organs can also undergo atrophy in response to the catabolic state.

Delayed healing: A prolonged catabolic state can compromise the body's ability to heal effectively.

Metabolic complications: These include hyperglycaemia, metabolic acidosis and other imbalances.

Interventions to counteract catabolism :

Nutrition: Adequate calorie and protein intake is crucial. Enteral nutrition, which involves feeding directly into the stomach or intestine via a tube, is often preferred.

Anabolic agents : Certain drugs can help counteract the catabolic effects, although their use requires careful evaluation.

Physical therapy: Early mobilisation and physiotherapy can help prevent excessive muscle loss.

Pain management: Good pain management can encourage food intake and mobilisation, thereby reducing catabolism.

Post-burn catabolism is a major challenge in the management of burn patients. Nurses and the medical team need to be vigilant and proactive in identifying signs of an increased catabolic state and intervening appropriately. Early and coordinated intervention is essential to improve patient outcomes and reduce the long-term complications associated with this condition.

Importance
enteral and parenteral nutrition

When it comes to caring for burn patients, nutrition plays a central role in the healing process. Energy and protein requirements increase dramatically after a severe burn due to the hypercatabolic metabolic response described above. Enteral nutrition (EN) and parenteral nutrition (PN) are two essential methods of meeting these needs.

Enteral nutrition (EN):

Definition: NE involves the administration of nutrients directly into the gastrointestinal tract via a tube, usually passed through the nose into the stomach (nasogastric tube) or the small intestine (nasojejunal tube).

Advantages :

Preserving intestinal integrity: Using the intestine helps to maintain its function and prevent atrophy of the intestinal wall.

Reduced risk of infection: Unlike NP, NE is associated with a lower risk of systemic infection.

Cost: Generally less expensive than NP.

Disadvantages and challenges :

Tolerance: Some patients may experience tolerance problems such as nausea, vomiting or diarrhoea.

Risk of aspiration: If the patient regurgitates, there is a risk of pulmonary aspiration.

Parenteral nutrition (NP):

Definition: NP is the administration of nutrients directly into the bloodstream via a central venous catheter.

Advantages :

Usefulness: Indicated for patients who cannot use their gastrointestinal tract or when NE is contraindicated.

Precise control: Intakes can be precisely adjusted to meet the patient's specific needs.

Disadvantages and challenges :

Risk of infection: NP may increase the risk of infections, particularly catheter-related infections.

Hepatic complications: Prolonged use of NP may lead to hepatic complications.

Cost: Generally more expensive than NE.

Considerations for burn patients :

Increased needs: Burn patients have significantly increased calorie and protein requirements to support healing and combat catabolism.

Regular assessment: It is essential to monitor nutrition regularly to ensure that the patient's needs are being met and to adjust intake as the patient progresses.

Nutrition, whether enteral or parenteral, is a cornerstone of care for burn patients. Nurses and the medical team must work closely with dieticians to develop and implement an appropriate nutritional plan, while closely monitoring the patient's condition and adjusting the plan as necessary.

Monitoring and adjustment energy needs

The nutritional management of burn patients is not static. Indeed, the energy needs of these patients evolve as their clinical condition changes. It is therefore essential to monitor their nutritional status closely and adjust energy intake accordingly.

The importance of monitoring :
Healing burns is an energy-intensive process, combined with the hypermetabolic response caused by the burn, so energy requirements are increased.

Inadequate nutrition can delay healing, increase the risk of infection, and have a negative impact on muscle function and mobility.

Initial assessment :
Calorie balance: Calculation of basic energy requirements, added to the additional requirements linked to the burn. Several formulas, such as Curreri's formula, can be used.

Protein balance: Proteins are essential for tissue repair. An adequate protein balance is also crucial.

Monitoring methods :
Body weight: Unexpected weight loss or gain may indicate an energy imbalance.

Nitrogen balance: Measurement of the quantity of nitrogen ingested in relation to that eliminated. A negative nitrogen balance suggests muscle breakdown.

Anthropometric measurements: such as skin fold or muscle circumference, to assess nutritional status.

Laboratory analyses: such as albumin and prealbumin, although their levels can be affected by factors other than nutrition.

Adjusting needs :

Reassessing needs: As the patient heals, the surface area of the burn decreases, reducing the need for additional calories.

Clinical responses: such as slow healing or signs of undernutrition, which suggest that nutritional intake needs to be adjusted.

Complications: Such as infections, which can increase energy requirements.

Level of activity: Mobilisation and rehabilitation increase energy expenditure.

Coordination with the medical team :

Monitoring and adjusting nutrition is a multidisciplinary task. Nurses, doctors, dieticians and therapists must work together to ensure optimal nutritional management.

Rigorous monitoring of burn patients' energy requirements and adjustment accordingly are essential to support healing, prevent complications and promote recovery. This is not a one-size-fits-all approach, but an individualised, ongoing assessment to meet the specific needs of each patient.

Chapter 6:
COMPLICATIONS
AND THEIR MANAGEMENT

Infections: Prevention and treatment

Burn patients are particularly vulnerable to infection due to the loss of the body's first line of defence: the skin. What's more, the inflammatory response associated with the burn, as well as the invasive procedures required for treatment, further increase this risk. Hence the vital importance of preventing and rapidly managing infections in these patients.

Why are burn patients at risk?

Compromised skin barrier: The skin acts as a barrier against pathogens. A burn destroys this barrier, leaving the underlying tissues exposed and vulnerable.

Immunosuppression: The immune response can be weakened after a burn, particularly as a result of stress, surgery and certain drugs.

Hospital environment: Prolonged stay in hospital exposes patients to nosocomial pathogens.

Infection prevention :

Rigorous hygiene: Hand washing is essential for care staff, patients and visitors.

Sterile care: Wounds must be cleaned, disinfected and dressed under sterile conditions.

Isolation: Depending on the severity of the burn and the patient's condition, isolation may be recommended.

46

Monitoring: Regular monitoring for signs of infection (redness, heat, pus, fever) is crucial.

Antibiotic prophylaxis: The use of antibiotics as a preventive measure may be considered in certain cases, although this is open to debate due to the risk of bacterial resistance.

Signs and symptoms of infection :

Local: Redness, heat, oedema, pus, delayed healing.

Systemic: fever, chills, tachycardia, hypotension.

Treatment of infections :

Identification of the pathogen: cultures taken to determine the causative agent and its sensitivity to antibiotics.

Antibiotic therapy: The choice of antibiotic should be based on the results of the cultures and adapted accordingly.

Haemodynamic support: In sepsis, maintaining arterial pressure and organ perfusion is crucial.

Surgical intervention: In some cases, surgical debridement of infected tissue is necessary.

Optimised wound care: Ensuring appropriate wound care to promote healing and reduce the bacterial load.

Bacterial resistance :

A growing challenge: Excessive use of antibiotics can lead to the emergence of resistant strains.

Preventive measures: Limit the use of antibiotics to what is strictly necessary, regularly monitor the patient's microbial flora and adopt rigorous sterile practices.

Preventing and managing infection in burn patients is a central aspect of their care. Constant vigilance, rapid response to signs of infection and close collaboration between the entire medical team are essential to minimise complications and optimise patient outcomes.

Healing:
Hypertrophy and contractures

When the skin suffers serious damage, as is the case with burns, the healing process is often accompanied by complications. Two of the most common complications following the healing of burns are hypertrophic scarring and contractures. These manifestations can have both functional and aesthetic consequences for the patient.

Hypertrophic scarring :
Definition: A hypertrophic scar is a thick, raised, reddish and often itchy scar that develops at the site of a previous wound. Unlike keloids, they generally do not extend beyond the boundaries of the original wound.

Risk factors: Tension on the wound, infection, delayed healing, location of the burn (certain areas of the body are more susceptible, such as the chest or joints).

Treatment: This may include massage, pressure dressings, steroid injections, cryotherapy, laser therapy and, in some cases, surgery.

Contractures :
Definition: Contractures are the result of shrinkage and hardening of skin, muscle or tendon tissue, which limits movement. In the context of burns, they often occur when a burn spreads over a joint.

Risk factors: Depth and extent of burn, location close to joints, prolonged immobilisation.

Treatment: Prevention is essential, hence the importance of early range-of-motion exercises and physiotherapy. If a contracture has already formed, treatment may require surgery to release the contracture, followed by rehabilitation.

Prevention :

Appropriate wound care: Proper wound care and debridement can reduce the risk of hypertrophic scarring.

Early mobilisation: Moving and stretching the burned area as soon as possible can prevent contractures from forming.

Sun protection: Healed skin is more sensitive to UV rays, which can worsen the appearance of scars. Sun protection is therefore recommended.

Psychological impact :

Scars and contractures are not just physical problems. They can have a significant impact on a patient's self-esteem, body image and overall quality of life.

It is essential to provide patients with psychological support, help them manage their new appearance and inform them about the treatment options available.

Hypertrophic scarring and contractures are potential but manageable complications of burns. With early intervention, multidisciplinary care and a focus on rehabilitation and prevention, many patients can return to normal function and improve the appearance of their scars. Care does not stop with wound closure; long-term support is often necessary to ensure the best possible outcome for burn patients.

Respiratory complications: Smoke inhalation and ventilation

Burns are not just skin lesions. In the event of fire or exposure to toxic fumes, the respiratory system can be seriously affected. Respiratory complications are among the most frequent causes of morbidity and mortality in burn patients, particularly in the first few hours and days following the incident.

Smoke inhalation :

Pathophysiology: Smoke inhalation causes inflammation and oedema of the respiratory tract, as well as a reduction in gas exchange capacity due to inhaled toxins.

Symptoms: Coughing, dyspnoea, wheezing, hoarseness and production of carbonaceous sputum.

Diagnosis: Bronchoscopy, pulse oximetry, arterial blood gas and thoracic imaging.

Treatment: oxygen therapy, bronchodilators, steroids and, in severe cases, intubation and mechanical ventilation.

Complications of inhalation :

Inhalation pneumonia: Infection of the lungs caused by inhaling bacteria from the mouth or throat.

Thermal damage: Direct heat damage can cause burns to the respiratory tract.

Carbon monoxide (CO) poisoning: This is a medical emergency in which CO displaces oxygen in the blood, causing hypoxia.

Mechanical ventilation :

Indications: Respiratory insufficiency, protection of the respiratory tract, or need for deep sedation for other treatments.

Mode and parameters: Depends on the severity of lung damage and the specific needs of the patient.

Possible complications: Barotrauma, pneumothorax, infections associated with ventilation.

Specific nursing care :

Monitoring: Regular monitoring of vital signs, oxygen saturation and ventilatory parameters.

Bronchial hygiene: Aspiration of secretions, use of mucolytic agents and respiratory physiotherapy.

Airway protection: Ensure that the endotracheal tube is securely fastened and that the head is in the neutral position to prevent accidental displacement or extubation.

Nutritional support: Patients on mechanical ventilation have increased energy requirements.

Respiratory rehabilitation :

Respiratory physiotherapy: Helps to mobilise secretions and improve lung function.

Breathing exercises: Like deep breathing techniques, to increase lung capacity.

Weaning off ventilation: A gradual process to enable the patient to resume independent breathing.

Respiratory complications following a burn can be severe and potentially fatal. Prompt and effective management of smoke inhalation and associated complications is essential for patient survival and recovery. The nurse's role in the monitoring, care and rehabilitation of these patients is central, requiring expertise, constant attention and close collaboration with the rest of the medical team.

Chapter 7:
REFURBISHMENT
AND PSYCHOSOCIAL SUPPORT

The rehabilitation process:
From hospital bed to home

The care of a burn patient does not end with the healing of their wounds. The consequences of a serious burn can last long after discharge from hospital, affecting both the physical function and the psychological well-being of the patient. Rehabilitation is therefore an essential part of the healing process.

Initial and ongoing assessment :
> **Physical:** Assessment of mobility, strength, endurance and functional limitations.
> **Psychological:** Assessment of mental health, self-esteem, body image and adaptation to trauma.
> **Social:** Consideration of support network, accommodation, employment and education needs.

Physical and occupational therapy :
> **Objectives:** Maintain and improve mobility, prevent contractures, strengthen muscles and make it easier to return to everyday activities.
> **Interventions:** Joint mobilisation, stretching, strengthening, occupational therapy and adapting daily activities.

Pain and scar management :
> **Physical therapy:** Techniques such as transcutaneous electrical stimulation (TENS) or ultrasound therapy.

Scar massage: Helps to reduce the thickness and hypersensitivity of scars.

Orthoses: Devices designed to immobilise or assist the movement of a joint or body segment.

Psychological support :

Individual therapy: Helps treat post-traumatic stress, depression, anxiety and other psychological disorders.

Support groups: to share experiences and coping strategies with other burn patients.

Education and training :

Self-care: Teaching scar care, sun protection and symptom management at home.

Vocational training: For those who need to adapt or change careers following injury.

Social reintegration and return to work :

Ability assessment: To determine whether the patient is capable of returning to their previous job or whether they need to be reoriented.

Job search support: Helping patients to find suitable work or to learn a new trade.

Long-term monitoring :

Burn follow-up clinics: Regular monitoring of scars, physical function and mental health.

Ongoing rehabilitation: Adjusting the rehabilitation plan as the patient's needs change.

Rehabilitation after a burn is a multi-dimensional, demanding and lengthy process. Each patient is unique, and their rehabilitation pathway needs to be tailored to their specific needs. With the right support, many burn patients can return to a full and meaningful life, overcoming the challenges imposed by their injury and the resulting scarring. The nurse's task is to accompany, guide and support the patient every step of the way, from the hospital bed to the home and beyond.

Supporting the patient:
Trauma management and psychological support

Suffering a serious burn is a deeply traumatic experience. Beyond the physical pain, the psychological after-effects can be just as devastating. Holistic care for burn patients must therefore include a psychological dimension, focusing on understanding, support and guidance.

The traumatic dimension of burns :
> **Initial shock:** The moment of the burn can feel like an attack, with a feeling of powerlessness and terror.
> **Pain:** This can be persistent, intense and cause significant distress.
> **Altered body image:** Disfigurement can lead to feelings of shame, embarrassment and isolation.

Common psychological reactions :
> **Post-traumatic stress disorder (PTSD):** Flashbacks, avoidance, neurovegetative hyperactivity.
> **Depression:** Sadness, apathy, loss of interest, suicidal thoughts.
> **Anxiety:** Agitation, heightened fears, sleep disorders.

Psychological assessment :
> **Clinical interviews:** to understand the patient's perceptions, fears and needs.
> **Questionnaires and scales:** Standardised tools for assessing the severity of symptoms.

Support strategies in the acute phase :

A reassuring presence: A simple presence, listening and touching can soothe.

Information: Explaining procedures, reassuring people about the next steps.

Relaxation techniques: deep breathing, meditation, soothing music.

Long-term therapies :

Cognitive-behavioural therapy: Helps patients to recognise and modify negative thoughts.

Exposure therapy: For patients with PTSD, getting them to gradually confront traumatic memories.

Art therapy and music therapy: A non-verbal way of expressing painful emotions.

Support groups :

Sharing experiences: Meeting other burn victims can reduce feelings of isolation.

Education: Experts can give advice on managing scars, body image and resuming daily life.

Family support :

Psychological support: Family members may also be traumatised or feel powerless.

Education: informing them on how best to help the patient, how to listen without being overprotective.

Preparing for discharge from hospital :

Anticipating: Preparing the patient to deal with the reactions of others and to answer sensitive questions.

Referrals: Refer patients to therapists or support groups appropriate to their situation.

Psychological support for burn patients is an essential part of their care. It involves not only guiding the patient through the challenges of pain and physical recovery, but also helping them to navigate the often turbulent waters of psychological trauma. Nurses, as the linchpin of patient care, play an essential role in this mission, always listening, always caring, providing both technical skills and humanity.

The importance of support groups and testimonials

When faced with the shocking ordeal of a serious burn, the healing process is not limited to a purely physical dimension. The trauma, altered body image and psychosocial consequences often lead to feelings of profound isolation. In this context, support groups and testimonials from other burn victims play an essential role in helping patients to rebuild their lives.

The power of the community :

Sense of belonging: Knowing that others have had similar experiences can reduce feelings of isolation.

A safe   environment: A space where patients can share without judgement or fear.

Support groups :

Structure and operation: Regular meetings, guided by professionals or peers.

A   wide range   of topics: pain management, body image acceptance, return to social and professional life.

Specific   workshops: For example, sessions on corrective make-up or scar management.

Testimonies :

A source of inspiration: Hearing how others have overcome similar challenges can be deeply motivating.

57

- **Diverse perspectives:** Each story is unique, offering a range of perspectives on healing and resilience.
- **Sharing platforms:** books, blogs, videos, live meetings.

Psychological benefits :
- **Validation:** Recognition of emotions and experiences.
- **Empowerment:** Reinforcing a sense of self-efficacy and mastery in the face of adversity.
- **Hope:** Seeing examples of success and reconstruction offers a positive outlook for the future.

Impact on family and friends :
- **Education:** Helping family and friends to understand the patient's experience.
- **Emotional support:** Offering family and friends a space to express their own feelings and concerns.
- **Support strategies:** Advice on how best to support their burn victim.

Limitations and precautions :
- **Don't force it:** Every patient is different, and not everyone is ready or willing to share in a group.
- **Managing group dynamics:** ensuring that the environment remains friendly and avoiding negative interactions.
- **Confidentiality:** Ensuring the protection of personal information and shared stories.

In the emotional and psychological maze that burn patients go through, the road to recovery is often tortuous. Support groups and testimonials act as compasses, offering guidance, encouragement and hope. They remind us that even in the darkest moments, human resilience can shine through, and that the community, with its stories of strength and courage, is there to light the way. For a nurse, encouraging these connections can often be the greatest gift given to a patient.

Chapter 8:
THE TECHNOLOGICAL ASPECT IN BURN CARE

The latest innovations in dressings and grafts

Medicine is a constantly evolving field, particularly when it comes to the treatment of burns. Recent advances in dressings and grafts have revolutionised the way we treat burn victims, offering a better chance of recovery, reduced pain and improved aesthetic results.

Hydrocolloid   dressings and hydrogels :

Moisture retention: These dressings maintain a moist environment, promoting healing and reducing pain.

Easy   to apply and remove: They can be removed without any additional trauma to the skin.

Panthenol and vitamin E dressings:

Stimulation of skin regeneration: These compounds promote skin healing by stimulating cell proliferation.

Scar reduction: They can help minimise the appearance of scars.

Artificial skin and skin substitutes :

Biomaterials: Use of collagen or silicone matrices to create a temporary or permanent structure over the wound.

Cell culture: The patient's own cells can be harvested, grown in the laboratory and then reapplied to the burn.

On-demand skin grafts :

3D printing: 3D printing technologies can now produce personalised skin grafts, using the patient's own cells to prevent rejection.

Bioreactors: These devices enable large areas of skin to be cultured for extensive grafts.

Stem cell transplants :

Regenerative potential: Stem cells taken from the patient or a donor can differentiate into various types of skin cells, speeding up healing.

Treatment of deep burns: These cells can help restore deeply damaged layers of skin.

Intelligent dressings :

Real-time monitoring: These dressings are equipped with sensors that can measure factors such as humidity, temperature and pH, providing valuable information about the condition of the wound.

Controlled drug delivery: Some intelligent dressings can release drugs or treatments in a targeted, controlled way.

Antimicrobial dressings :

Silver and honey: These natural substances have antimicrobial properties and are incorporated into dressings to prevent infection.

Antimicrobial peptides: These synthetic molecules can target and destroy specific bacteria, offering personalised protection against infection.

Innovations in dressings and grafts illustrate the ingenuity and determination of researchers to improve care for burn patients. For nurses, these advances represent new tools and techniques to ensure the best possible care. While science continues to evolve, the objective remains constant: to enable rapid, effective healing that respects the patient's well-being.

Use of telemedicine for remote monitoring

At a time when technology is increasingly present in all aspects of our lives, medicine is no exception to this transformation. Telemedicine, or the use of information and communication technologies to provide medical care at a distance, has begun to play a major role in the follow-up of burn patients, revolutionising the way in which these patients are cared for after leaving hospital.

Introduction to telemedicine :
Definition: Use of technology to provide remote medical care.
History: From modest beginnings to current applications in almost every medical field.
The benefits of telemedicine for burn patients :
Easier access: For those who live far from specialist centres, telemedicine eliminates the need for frequent travel.
Reduced costs: less travel, fewer days in hospital.
Regular monitoring: Allows regular observation of the progress of the burn, facilitating early intervention in the event of complications.
Patient comfort: Follow-up is carried out in the comfort of their own home.
Practical details:
Dedicated platforms : Applications and websites designed specifically for telemedicine.

Video consultations: real-time interaction between patient and healthcare professional.

Medical photography: Used to visually assess the condition of the burn and monitor its progress.

Secure data transmission: All information is exchanged using secure protocols to guarantee confidentiality.

The role of the nurse in telemedicine :

Education: Teaching patients how to use telemedicine tools.

Regular check-ups: Plan and carry out regular check-ups via online platforms.

Interpretation: Helping to decipher and analyse the information provided by the patient.

Challenges and concerns :

Technological limitations: Not all patients have access to suitable technology or a stable Internet connection.

Training: Ensure that medical staff are trained in telemedicine tools.

Legal and ethical aspects: guaranteeing data confidentiality and security, obtaining the patient's informed consent.

Case studies and testimonials :

Concrete examples: How telemedicine has improved the care of certain patients.

Testimonials: The personal experiences of patients and healthcare professionals using telemedicine.

As telemedicine continues to evolve, its value in monitoring burn patients is becoming increasingly clear. It offers a practical, cost-effective and patient-centred solution for ensuring regular, high-quality medical follow-up. For nurses, it represents an extension of their role, enabling them to provide ongoing care while strengthening the link with the patient, even at a distance. By adopting and adapting these technological innovations, the nursing profession is helping to shape the future of medical care.

The role of simulation in training: reproducing real-life situations

Simulation in medical training is an educational approach that uses equipment, devices and/or virtual environments to reproduce real or potential situations. In the context of burn care, simulation offers an invaluable opportunity to train nurses and medical teams to respond to complex situations in a controlled environment.

Introduction to medical simulation :

Origins: From aeronautical training to medicine.

Development : The rise of simulation technologies and their integration into the medical curriculum.

Types of simulation :

High-fidelity mannequins: Anatomically correct models capable of reproducing vital signs and symptoms.

Virtual simulations: Computer programmes and augmented reality to immerse students in a medical situation.

Role-playing: staging scenarios with actors playing the role of patients.

Benefits of simulation :

Risk-free practice: Learners can make mistakes with no real consequences for the patient.

Reproduction of rare scenarios: Simulate infrequent but serious situations requiring a rapid and effective response.

Immediate feedback: Trainers can offer real-time feedback and debriefings after each session.

Confidence-building: Exposure to repeated situations strengthens learners' skills and confidence.

Application in the management of burns:

Initial assessment: Simulating the arrival of a severely burned patient.

Airway management: Training in the management of respiratory complications in burn victims.

Invasive procedures: Performing techniques such as debridement or skin grafting on mannequins.

Emotional management: role-playing situations to help carers manage their emotions and those of their patients.

Integrating simulation into the curriculum :

Initial training: Include simulation from the earliest stages of nurse training.

Ongoing training: Regular refresher courses to update and reinforce skills.

Challenges and prospects :

High cost: High-tech simulation can be expensive.

Technological updating: Keeping equipment and programmes up to date.

Training the trainers: Ensuring that trainers are competent to teach using simulation.

Validation: Ongoing research to demonstrate the effectiveness of simulation in improving patient outcomes.

Simulation training has radically transformed the way nurses and medical teams are prepared to meet the challenges of burn care. It replicates the stress, urgency and complexity of real-life situations while providing a safe learning environment. As technology continues to advance, it is certain that simulation will play an increasingly central role in the training of healthcare professionals, preparing them optimally to provide quality care to burn patients.

Chapter 9:
ETHICS AND BURN CARE

Informed consent
and respect for patient autonomy

Informed consent is a cornerstone of modern medicine, reflecting the intrinsic value placed on patient autonomy. In the context of burn treatment, where interventions can be invasive, painful and have long-term implications, the importance of informed consent and respect for autonomy cannot be underestimated.

Understanding informed   consent :
> **Background:** From simple authorisation to an information exchange process.
> **Ethical principles:** Autonomy, beneficence, non-maleficence and justice.
> **Legislation:** The laws and regulations in force concerning medical consent.

Elements of informed consent :
> **Information:** Patients must be fully informed about their condition, the treatment options available and the associated risks and benefits.
> **Understanding:** Patients must understand the information provided, avoiding medical jargon.
> **Willingness:** Consent must be given voluntarily, without coercion or pressure.
> **Capacity:** The patient must be mentally and emotionally capable of making a decision.

The importance of dialogue :
> **Active listening:** Paying attention to the patient's concerns, questions and values.

Questioning: Encourage patients to ask questions to clarify their doubts.

Adaptability: Adapting information to the patient's level of understanding and specific needs.

Consent in the context of burns :

Emergency versus autonomy: Navigating situations where rapid treatment is required, while respecting the patient's autonomy.

Special considerations: Patients under the influence of medication, children or traumatised individuals may require adapted approaches to consent.

Refusal of treatment :

Respect the decision: Even if the medical staff do not agree.

Counselling: Offering guidance and support in the event of refusal, to ensure that the patient fully understands the implications.

Special cases :

Legal guardians: For patients incapable of giving consent (children, people with cognitive impairment).

Emergency situations: When there is no time to obtain full informed consent.

Challenges and concerns :

Language barriers: How to ensure informed consent when the patient and the healthcare professional do not speak the same language.

Cultural diversity: Respecting and understanding different cultural perspectives on health and treatment.

Informed consent is much more than a mere administrative formality; it is a manifestation of the profound respect accorded to the patient's autonomy and dignity. In the treatment of burns, where decisions can have lifelong consequences, this balance between providing optimal care and respecting the patient's wishes is both an art and a science. It is a constant reminder to healthcare professionals of the intrinsic humanity of their work, affirming that each patient is not only a body to be cared for, but also a voice to be listened to and a will to be respected.

Reflections on the end of life on relentless treatment

The management of severely burned patients confronts medical teams with major ethical dilemmas. One of the most poignant is the balance between prolonging life through intensive medical intervention and recognising that there may be times when limiting or stopping treatment may be in the patient's best interests. This chapter looks at the delicate issue of therapeutic prolongation at the end of life.

Understanding therapeutic overkill :
Definition: Distinction between legitimate intensive care and excessive treatment with no real benefit for the patient.
Background: The development of medical technologies and the ability to prolong life.
Ethical principles at stake :
Autonomy: Respect for the patient's wishes and values.
Beneficence: Providing optimal well-being for the patient.
Non-maleficence: Doing no harm or avoiding causing unnecessary harm.
Justice: Ensuring fairness in decision-making.

Assessment of quality of life :

- **Inherent challenges:** The subjectivity of the notion of "quality of life".
- **Clinical evaluation:** To assess the potential for functional recovery, pain and other morbidities.
- **Patient perspective:** how the patient perceives their quality of life and future expectations.

Communication with the patient and family :

- **Openness:** Encouraging honest dialogue about prognosis and treatment options.
- **Emotional support:** Recognising and responding to the emotional needs of patients and their families.
- **Shared decision-making:** actively involving the patient and family in decisions about care.

Decision to limit or stop treatment :

- **Clinical considerations:** Analyse the chances of recovery and the potential benefits of interventions.
- **Ethical considerations:** Evaluate whether continued care constitutes therapeutic overkill.
- **Advance directives :** The importance of advance directives drawn up by the patient.

Support at the end of life :

- **Palliative care:** relieving pain and improving quality of life.
- **Psychological support:** for the patient, the family and the care team.
- **Ritual and spirituality:** Recognising the importance of spiritual needs at the end of life.

Reflection on the role of carers:

- **Emotional challenges:** Dealing with stress, guilt and bereavement.
- **Professional support: the** importance of supervision, discussion groups and ongoing training.

The end of life is a delicate moment, requiring sensitivity, compassion and wisdom on the part of carers. In the care of patients with severe burns, it is crucial to recognise when the fight for life can turn into therapeutic overkill, no longer serving the patient's well-being. These reflections on the end of life are a reminder of the importance of human dignity and respect for each individual, even in the darkest and most complex moments of medicine.

The cultural dimension: respect for beliefs and traditional practices

The management of patients in the burns context, as in any other medical field, must be imbued with cultural sensitivity. Cultural and religious beliefs can influence perceptions of illness, treatment decisions and the way in which patients and their families experience medical care. In this section, we explore how the cultural dimension intertwines with medical care.

Introduction to cultural competence :

Definition: What is cultural competence in healthcare?

Importance: Why is it essential in the treatment of burn victims?

Recognising the diversity of beliefs surrounding burns :

Origins of burns: How different cultures perceive the cause of burns.

Treatment and healing: The various traditional approaches and beliefs associated with the healing process.

Intercultural communication :

Language barriers: The importance of interpreters and accurate translations.

Unspoken words and nuances: Recognising that communication goes beyond words.

Active listening: A key to truly understanding the patient's perspective.

Respectful integration of traditional practices :

Assessment of practices: Determining whether they are complementary or potentially harmful.

Dialogue: Openly discuss concerns while valuing the patient's beliefs.

Accommodations: Where possible and safe, incorporate traditional remedies or rituals into the care plan.

Religious considerations :

Rituals: Taking into account ritual needs, such as prayers or purification rites.

Perspectives on suffering and death: how different religions approach these concepts and how this can influence medical decisions.

Ethics and end-of-life decisions :

Respect for values: Every culture has its own vision of life, death, dignity and suffering.

Informed consent: Ensuring that the patient and family truly understand, in their cultural context, the implications of medical decisions.

Family support :

Family roles: In some cultures, the family plays a central role in medical decisions.

Mourning and funeral rites: Understanding and respecting the diverse ways in which cultures experience mourning and honour the dead.

Modern medicine, with its technological advances, must also be deeply rooted in humanity. Respecting the cultural dimension of care is a way of affirming the dignity and uniqueness of each patient. By bridging the gap between medical knowledge and cultural beliefs, carers can offer truly patient-centred and holistic care, reflecting a deeply empathetic and respectful approach to medicine.

Chapter 10:
THE IMPORTANCE OF PREVENTION

Public education:
Campaigns and awareness-raising

Educating the public about the risks and prevention of burns is of paramount importance. Throughout the ages, communities have faced dangers from fire, boiling water, chemicals and electricity. But despite the constant challenges, humanity has always had the capacity to adapt, learn and grow. As a result, awareness and education campaigns have become a cornerstone in protecting society from potential dangers.

From childhood, we learn to fear and respect fire. Tales and legends handed down from generation to generation have often served as warnings. But as society evolves, education methods must also adapt. Today, thanks to the media and technology, we have the opportunity to reach millions of people, share poignant stories and offer practical advice on how to prevent burns.

Awareness campaigns are not just about prevention. They also provide resources for those who have suffered burns, highlighting stories of survival, resilience and hope. Through these campaigns, society is informed of the challenges faced by survivors, their struggles, but also their triumphs.

But for a campaign to be effective, it must be relevant and resonate with its audience. It must use a variety of communication methods, such as social media, television, radio and community workshops. Each message must be tailored to its audience, whether they are children playing near a cooker, workers on a building site or elderly people living alone.

As well as media campaigns, community engagement is essential. Organising workshops, demonstrations and educational programmes in schools, community centres and workplaces can have a profound impact. Direct interaction not only allows information to be shared, but also allows concerns to be addressed, personal stories to be heard and future programmes to be tailored to the needs of the community.

However, public education is not just about prevention and support. It also aims to break down the stigma associated with burns. By sharing stories of survival, demonstrating medical advances and celebrating the diversity of human experience, we can help to create a more understanding and empathetic society.

Ultimately, education and awareness are powerful tools to protect, guide and unite the community. Through effective communication, sincere community involvement and a dedication to lifelong learning, we can not only prevent burns, but also support those affected and build a safer, more caring world for all.

Advice
to avoid accidents in the home

The home is often perceived as a sanctuary, a place of safety and comfort. However, many accidents occur in the home. While some of these incidents may be minor, others can have serious or even fatal consequences. Fortunately, many domestic accidents can be avoided through prevention and awareness. Here are some tips on how to ensure a safe home environment for everyone.

Falls prevention :

Make staircases safe: Use child safety gates and install sturdy handrails.

Remove obstacles: Make sure aisles and corridors are clear. Avoid leaving objects lying around.

Secure the carpets: Use non-slip pads to prevent the carpets from slipping.

Lighting: Make sure your home is well lit, especially areas such as staircases.

Prevention of burns :

Cooking: Never leave the handles of saucepans facing outwards and use rear lights wherever possible.

Hot water: Set the water heater to a maximum temperature of 50°C.

Chemical products: Keep household products out of the reach of children.

Preventing poisoning:

Medicines: Keep all medicines in childproof containers and out of their reach.

Chemical products: Always read labels and store hazardous products away from food.

Drowning prevention :

Swimming pools: Install a barrier with a lockable door around swimming pools. Never leave children unsupervised near water.

Bathrooms: Never leave a child unsupervised in a bathtub, even one with little water.

Protection against electricity :

Sockets: Use protectors for electrical sockets if you have young children.

Cables: Do not overload sockets and keep cables away from passageways.

Fire protection :

Detectors: Install smoke and carbon monoxide detectors and check their operation regularly.

Evacuation plan: Draw up a fire evacuation plan and practise it with all family members.

Candles: Never leave a burning candle unattended.

Child safety :

Entrapment: Avoid furniture with spaces where children can get their heads or fingers stuck.

Toxic products: Keep cleaning products, pesticides and similar products out of the reach of children.

Pet safety :

Make sure your houseplants are not toxic to animals.

Avoid leaving small objects lying around that animals could swallow.

By taking these precautions and being constantly vigilant, many domestic accidents can be avoided. A safe home is one where every member of the family, from the youngest to the oldest, can live and thrive without fear of unexpected accidents.

Integration of prevention programmes in schools

School plays a central role in the lives of children and teenagers. It is not only a place of academic learning, but also a place where young people acquire essential life skills. Integrating prevention programmes into schools is therefore an effective strategy for reaching large numbers of young people and raising their awareness of various safety issues. Here's how it can be done:

- Needs assessment :
    - Before implementing a prevention programme, it is essential to identify the specific needs of the school. This can be done through surveys of pupils, parents and teachers, or by analysing past incidents.
- Programme development :
    - Once the needs have been identified, it's time to develop a tailored programme. This could include workshops, demonstrations, simulations, specific courses or presentations by professionals.
- Teacher training :
    - To ensure the effectiveness of the programme, it is crucial that teachers are well trained to deliver it. They should receive regular training to keep abreast of best practice and new findings.
- Curricular integration :
    - Incorporate prevention lessons into the existing curriculum. For example, science lessons can cover the dangers of chemical products, while sports lessons can deal with safety during physical activities.
- Interactive activities :
    - Young people are often more receptive when learning is interactive. Organise practical workshops, games, simulations or competitions to make the subject more engaging.
- Involvement of parents :
    - Parents play an essential role in prevention. Organise information meetings to make them aware of potential dangers and provide advice on how to improve safety at home.

- Community partnerships :
  - Work with the local police, fire brigade, hospitals and other relevant organisations to increase the programme's reach and impact.
- Continuous assessment and improvement :
  - Once the programme has been implemented, it is essential to evaluate its effectiveness. Gather feedback, analyse incidents and adapt the programme accordingly.
- Promoting a culture of prevention :
  - Encourage a culture where safety is valued. This could include recognising students who demonstrate safe behaviour or setting up a school safety club.
- Regular updates :
  - Society is changing, and so are the potential dangers facing young people. Make sure you update the programme regularly to keep it relevant.

By integrating prevention programmes into schools, we are giving young people a solid foundation on which to build a secure future. It is essential to recognise that prevention is a community effort that requires the commitment and collaboration of everyone to ensure the well-being of our children.

Chapter 11:
THE CHALLENGES OF THE HOSPITAL ENVIRONMENT

Resource management: human, material and financial

Effective resource management is essential to the smooth running and success of any organisation, whether it's a hospital, a business or a school. The judicious allocation of human, material and financial resources not only ensures smooth operations, but also maximises productivity and profitability.

1. Human resources :

Strategic planning: Identify current and future staffing needs to meet organisational objectives.

Recruitment and selection: Put in place robust processes to attract and select the right talent.

Training and development: Ensure that staff are well trained and have the necessary skills to meet the demands of their jobs.

Performance evaluation: Setting up regular evaluation systems to measure performance and identify areas for improvement.

Employee well-being: Satisfied, healthy employees are more productive. Invest in the well-being of your staff.

2. Material resources :

Needs assessment: Regularly assess the organisation's material needs.

Procurement: Acquire the equipment you need wisely, looking for quality and cost-effectiveness.

Maintenance: Make sure that all equipment and installations are well maintained to avoid interruptions.

Inventory: Keep an accurate record of all material assets to track usage, depreciation and eventual replacement.

Security: Protect your hardware resources against theft, damage and other losses.

3. Financial resources :

Budgeting: Draw up a clear budget detailing expected income and planned expenditure.

Expense tracking: Keep accurate records of expenses to ensure they remain within budget.

Risk management: Identify and assess potential financial risks and put in place measures to mitigate them.

Reporting: Create regular financial reports to inform decision-makers and stakeholders of the organisation's financial health.

Investments : For surplus funds, consider sound investments that can offer future returns.

Cost optimisation: Look for ways to optimise costs while maintaining or improving the quality of services or products.

Each type of resource presents its own challenges and requires special attention. Effective resource management requires strategic planning, continuous monitoring and adaptability to meet the changing needs of the organisation. Ultimately, the aim is to use these resources in a way that maximises value for the organisation while ensuring its long-term sustainability.

Ensuring quality of care
in a stressful environment

Working in the medical field, and particularly in a specialist service such as a burns unit, requires not only clinical expertise, but also the ability to function effectively in an often stressful environment. The challenges are many: the severity of cases, the emotional needs of patients and their families, and the constant pressure to provide quality care. Here's how to ensure quality care while managing the stress of the environment:

1. Continuing education :
Medicine is constantly evolving. To provide the best possible care, it is essential to keep up to date with the latest techniques, treatments and research. Regular training can help healthcare professionals feel more competent and less stressed in the face of daily challenges.

2. Clear protocols :
Having clear guidelines and protocols in place ensures that, even in stressful situations, staff know exactly what action to take. This minimises errors and ensures continuity of care.

3. Team support :
Cultivate a supportive working environment. Teams that work well together can share workloads, offer advice and reduce feelings of isolation.

4. Supervision and feedback :
Regular supervision and feedback sessions help to identify potential problems early on, reinforce good practice and provide a forum for discussing concerns.

5. Stress reduction measures :
Introduce stress management techniques such as meditation, breathing exercises or regular breaks to help staff recharge during the day.

6. Psychological support services :
Recognise the emotional impact of working in a stressful environment. Offer access to counselling or psychological support for those who need it.

7. Morbidity and mortality reviews :
Hold regular meetings to review cases where results were less than optimal. This provides an opportunity to learn, adjust practices and continually improve care.

8. Patient involvement :
Actively involve patients and their families in decisions about their care. This creates a care partnership and can contribute to greater patient satisfaction.

9. Technology and innovation :
Use technology to improve the quality of care, whether through electronic medical records for better coordination of care or innovations that directly improve treatment.

10. Staff development :
Regularly recognise and reward staff for their dedication and hard work. Valued staff are more likely to stay engaged and motivated.
Ultimately, the key to ensuring quality care in a stressful environment lies in a combination of solid training, robust support and open communication. When these elements are in place, even the most stressful challenges can be tackled with skill and care.

Liaison with other hospital departments (intensive care, surgery, etc.)

The care of patients, particularly those with severe burns, often requires a multidisciplinary approach. The burns service does not operate in isolation; it works closely with other hospital services to ensure holistic care. Understanding and optimising this liaison is essential for effective treatment.

1. The importance of collaboration :

The complex nature of severe burns can involve complications that are beyond the remit of a single department. For example, a severely burned patient may require intensive care, reconstructive surgery, respiratory assistance or psychological support.

2. Resuscitation :

Burn patients, particularly those with burns over a large part of their body, may require resuscitation to stabilise their vital functions. Close collaboration with the intensive care unit ensures a smooth transition for patients between departments.

3. Surgery :

The burn unit and the surgical department need to work hand in hand, especially when it comes to procedures such as surgical debridement, skin grafts or reconstructive surgery. Fluid communication between these teams is essential to the successful planning and execution of these procedures.

4. Pneumology :

Patients who have inhaled smoke or toxic gases may have respiratory lesions that require intervention by the Respiratory Department. Assessment and treatment of lung damage is often an essential component of recovery.

5. Dermatology :

As well as treating burns immediately, dermatologists can play a crucial role in the healing phase and preventing unsightly or debilitating scars.

6. Psychiatry and psychology :

The trauma associated with a severe burn is not just physical. Victims may suffer from post-traumatic stress disorder, anxiety, depression or other mental disorders. Appropriate psychological care is therefore essential.

7. Physiotherapy :

Post-burn rehabilitation is vital to maintain mobility and minimise contractions. Physiotherapists help with the patient's physical rehabilitation.

8. Nutrition :

The energy requirements of burn patients are significantly increased. Dieticians can therefore be called upon to develop appropriate diets.

9. Case management and social workers :

Navigating through convalescence can be a challenge for patients and their families. Case managers and social workers can offer valuable support by coordinating care and providing resources.

10. Interdepartmental communication :

One crucial point is to ensure transparent and regular communication between the various departments. Multidisciplinary meetings, where cases are discussed collectively, can facilitate this collaboration.

Each hospital department brings its own unique expertise, and their harmonious integration is essential to offer burn patients the best chance of recovery and a return to a normal life.

CHAPTER 12:
BACK TO THE COMPANY
AND SELF-ACCEPTANCE

Aesthetic reconstruction: reconstructive surgery and medical tattooing

Once the acute phase of a burn has been managed and healing begins, a new phase begins for many patients: that of aesthetic reconstruction. This phase is crucial, as it has profound implications not only for the patient's physical appearance, but also for their emotional and psychological well-being.

1. Reconstructive surgery :
After burns, the skin may contract, leaving stretched or deformed areas. The aim of reconstructive surgery is to restore function and improve the aesthetic appearance of these areas. It may involve techniques such as :
- **Z-plasties:** Z-shaped incisions are used to reorganise or redistribute skin tension.
- **Lambeaux:** Pieces of tissue, with their blood supply, are moved to cover a defect area.
- **Skin expansion:** Uses balloons inserted under the skin to gradually stretch healthy skin, which can then be used to cover a neighbouring area.

2. Medical tattoo :
Medical tattooing, or micropigmentation, is a technique that involves the insertion of pigments into the dermis to improve the appearance of burn scars. It can help to :

- **Camouflage scars:** Pigments are chosen to match the patient's natural skin colour, reducing the appearance of scars.
- **Restore facial features:** If a burn has affected areas such as the eyebrows or lips, medical tattooing can help redefine these areas.

3. Dermabrasion and chemical peels :
These techniques aim to remove or reduce the superficial layers of skin to improve the texture and appearance of burn scars.

4. Laser therapy :
Lasers can be used to improve the colour, texture and elasticity of scars. They can also help to reduce the redness or pigmentation of scars.

5. The role of psychology :
Cosmetic reconstruction is not just about looking good. Patients may have complex or ambivalent feelings about surgery or feel anxious about its outcome. Psychological support is essential to help them navigate these emotions and make informed decisions.

6. Time and patience :
Aesthetic reconstruction is often a lengthy process, which may require several surgical procedures and non-surgical treatments over several years. Patients need to be informed about this journey and realistic expectations need to be set.

Aesthetic reconstruction after a severe burn is a journey that combines the art and science of medicine. Although the road can be long and sometimes difficult, modern advances offer hope of significant improvement, both functionally and aesthetically, for burn survivors.

The role of associations of burn victims

When people are seriously burned, they face not only physical challenges, but also emotional, psychological and social ones. Burn victims' associations play an indispensable role in bridging the gap between initial medical care and a return to a full and rewarding life. They act as a support network, providing valuable resources for burn victims and their families.

1. Emotional and psychological support :
Associations often organise support groups for survivors. These groups enable victims to share their experiences, discuss their challenges and find comfort in the company of people who have been in similar situations.

2. Education :
Associations educate survivors about burn healing, pain management, reconstructive surgery and other aspects of recovery. This information can help patients understand their situation and make informed decisions about their care.

3. Advocacy :
Many associations defend the rights of burn victims, ensuring that the policies and laws in place fully support their recovery and reintegration into society.

4. Raising awareness :
As well as providing support for victims, the associations also play a crucial role in raising public awareness of the dangers that can lead to burns and how to prevent these accidents.

5. Camps for children :

Associations often organise therapeutic camps for young survivors. These camps allow children to find themselves, learn life skills and boost their self-esteem in a safe and stimulating environment.

6. Financial assistance :

Some associations may offer financial assistance or resources to help burn victims cover the costs of treatment, equipment or adaptations needed at home.

7. Resources for rehabilitation :

They also provide information on rehabilitation centres, therapists and other medical professionals specialising in the treatment of burns.

8. Forums and workshops :

These events enable survivors, families and professionals to meet and exchange knowledge, experience and best practice.

9. Support for research :

Numerous associations support research into burn treatments, reconstructive surgery and innovative therapies, in the hope of bringing about continuous improvements in burns care.

Burn victims' associations play a multifaceted role, encompassing both patient support and public awareness. Their work, often fuelled by passion and empathy, is an essential component of the burns care ecosystem.

Helping patients to find their place again: professional, social and family support

Healing from a serious burn goes far beyond physical restoration. The scar, whether visible or hidden, can profoundly affect a person's identity, sense of belonging and ability to interact with the outside world. It is a journey that requires a holistic approach, focusing on professional, social and family rehabilitation.

1. Professional support :
   - **Training and rehabilitation:** Workshops can be organised to help victims acquire new skills or adapt their existing skills to new professional roles.
   - **Career counselling:** Specialists can guide patients through career options suited to their new reality.
   - **Workplace adaptations:** Ensuring the necessary adaptations, such as flexible working hours, an ergonomic environment or access to medical devices.

2. Social support :
   - **Group therapy:** These sessions offer patients a space to share their experiences, fears and hopes with others who have been through similar experiences.
   - **Social and leisure activities:** These encourage interaction and rebuild self-confidence. Taking part in activities such as sport, art or music can be particularly therapeutic.
   - **Awareness-raising events:** Taking part in events that raise awareness of burn trauma can give meaning to their experience and help reduce stigma.

3. Family support :
   - **Family therapy:** Burns to a limb can change family dynamics. Therapy helps to resolve tensions, clarify roles and strengthen bonds.

- **Training for carers:** Family members may need training to assist the patient with their daily routine or medical care.
- **Sharing spaces for relatives:** Support groups for relatives can help them to manage their own stress and better support the patient.

4. Community integration :
- **Mentoring programmes:** Former patients can act as mentors for new patients, providing them with a unique and reassuring perspective.
- **Liaison with community services:** This ensures that patients have access to services such as adapted transport, assistance programmes or housing initiatives.

5. Self-esteem support :
- **Image advice:** Teaching patients to use clothing or make-up to manage the visibility of scars can improve their confidence.
- **Individual psychological support:** Individual therapy can help address issues of self-esteem, body shaming or identity.

The road to a full life after a serious burn is an arduous one. However, with the right support covering professional, social and family dimensions, a patient can not only heal, but thrive, regain their place in society and lead a rich and fulfilling life.

Chapter 13:
CONTINUING TRAINING
AND RESEARCH

Conferences and webinars
and workshops to follow

In the medical field, and particularly in the care of patients with severe burns, continuing education is essential if we are to remain at the cutting edge of knowledge and practice. Healthcare professionals need to be up to date with new techniques, innovative research and best practice to offer patients the best possible care. Conferences, webinars and workshops are excellent ways of learning, networking and exchanging knowledge.

1. Conferences :
   - **International congresses:** These events bring together experts from all over the world. They offer an overview of advances in burn care and provide an opportunity for fruitful exchanges between professionals.
   - **National conferences:** These more localised events provide an opportunity to address issues specific to a given region or population.

2. Webinars :
   - **Educational series:** Some organisations or associations offer educational series on specific subjects, enabling professionals to expand their knowledge without having to travel.
   - **Presentations of recent research :** Rapid dissemination of new discoveries is essential in the

92

medical field. Webinars are an excellent way of sharing these advances in real time.

3. Workshops :
- **Practical workshops:** These are interactive sessions where participants can practise new techniques under the supervision of experts. Topics may include pain management, dressing techniques or reconstructive surgery.
- **Clinical simulations:** These workshops enable professionals to simulate real-life clinical scenarios to hone their skills.

How do you choose the right events?
- **Examine the speakers:** Finding out who the guest experts are and what they will be talking about can give you an idea of the event's relevance to your professional practice.
- **Read the reviews:** feedback from other professionals can help determine whether the event is relevant and of high quality.
- **Consider the logistics:** Although content is crucial, you also need to consider the costs, location and format of the event (in person, online, hybrid).

Conferences, webinars and workshops play a vital role in the continuing education of healthcare professionals. For those working with burn patients, these events offer a unique opportunity to immerse themselves in advances in the field, exchange ideas with peers and strengthen their skills to improve the quality of care offered to patients.

The importance of clinical research: advances and discoveries

Clinical research is the driving force behind all medical advances. It allows us to acquire new knowledge, develop new treatments and improve existing protocols. In the field of burns, the importance of clinical research is all the more crucial, as it offers the promise of faster healing, less invasive techniques, less pain and a better quality of life for patients.

1. Why is clinical research essential?
- **Understanding the mechanisms of burns:** Research is helping to improve our understanding of the physiological, immunological and cellular reactions that occur when a burn is sustained.
- **Evaluating treatments:** Thanks to research, it is possible to evaluate the effectiveness and safety of new treatments, drugs or surgical techniques.
- **Personalised approaches:** Every patient is unique, and clinical research aims to develop tailor-made treatments adapted to the specific needs of each individual.

2. Recent advances thanks to clinical research :
- **Skin grafts:** The development of advanced skin grafting techniques, including the use of laboratory-grown skin, has revolutionised the treatment of burn victims.
- **Pain management:** The study of new analgesics and non-medicinal methods, such as virtual reality, has led to better management of patients' pain.
- **Intelligent dressings:** These dressings, impregnated with antibiotics or capable of monitoring wound hydration, offer more precise monitoring and better healing.

3. Promising discoveries on the horizon :
- **Cell therapy:** The use of stem cells to regenerate damaged tissue is a fast-growing field.

- **Nanotechnology:** The use of nanoparticles to deliver drugs directly to the wound or to create dressings with unique properties has great potential.
- **Bioprinting:** 3D printing of skin tissue is a fascinating avenue of research, with the possibility of creating tailor-made grafts for each patient.

4. The challenges of clinical research :
- **Ethics:** All clinical trials must be conducted in accordance with ethical principles, guaranteeing the safety and well-being of patients.
- **Funding:** Research requires resources, and funding remains a major challenge, despite the vital importance of clinical research.
- **Adopting new methods:** Integrating advances in research into everyday clinical practice requires time and resources.

Clinical research is inextricably linked to developments in the care of patients with severe burns. Every discovery and advance offers a glimmer of hope to patients who are often faced with intense pain and considerable challenges in their healing process. It is thanks to research that medicine continues to progress, to innovate and to improve the lives of those who depend on it.

Publications and specialist journals: keeping up to date

In the dynamic world of medicine, healthcare professionals are constantly confronted with new information. Medical discoveries, technological advances and changes in clinical recommendations occur at a rapid pace. For a nurse or any other professional working in the field of burns, keeping up to date is not only essential to ensuring quality care, it is also an ethical obligation. This is where specialist publications and journals come in.

1. Why are specialist publications crucial?
- **Updating knowledge:** Journals provide an overview of the latest research, enabling professionals to learn about new techniques, therapies or medicines.
- **Peer validation:** Studies published in specialist journals are generally subjected to a peer review process, which guarantees the quality and reliability of the information.
- **Interprofessional exchanges:** These enable experts to share their experiences, learn from each other and work together to improve patient care.

2. Some key journals in the field of burns :
- **"Burns":** This international journal covers all aspects of burns, from basic research to clinical care.
- **"Journal of Burn Care & Research:** provides information on the latest advances in burn care and rehabilitation.
- **"Annals of Burns and Fire Disasters":** focusing on fire-related disasters and their medical consequences.

3. How can the new information be integrated into daily practice?
- **Continuing education:** Workshops, seminars and conferences based on recent articles enable new knowledge to be integrated directly into clinical practice.
- **Discussion groups:** Regular meetings with colleagues to discuss the latest publications can stimulate enriching exchanges and practical applications.
- **Modern technologies:** digital applications and platforms now offer summaries, analyses and

comments on recent articles, making it easier to access and understand information.

4. The challenges ahead :
  - **Volume of information:** The abundance of new publications can be overwhelming. It's essential to learn how to filter and prioritise information.
  - **Constructive criticism:** Not every article or study is clinically relevant. Professionals need to develop a critical mind to assess the validity and applicability of information.

Specialist publications and journals are a cornerstone of continuing medical education. They represent a bridge between clinical research and the day-to-day reality of the patient. For nurses and all healthcare professionals, engaging in regular, critical reading of these journals is an essential step in ensuring evidence-based care and meeting patients' needs as effectively as possible.

Chapter 14:
TESTIMONIALS AND CASE STUDIES

Challenges and victories:
nurses' stories

Let's delve into the heart of the burns unit, where every day is a mixture of intense challenges and personal and professional triumphs. Behind every dressing, every infusion, lies a human story. Through the stories of the nurses, discover the daily lives of these behind-the-scenes heroes who fight with passion and dedication for their patients.

1. Sarah: The importance of the first hour
Sarah recounts her first experience with a patient who has suffered burns to more than 60% of his body. The first hour is often referred to as the "Golden Hour", as it is the moment when rapid intervention can make all the difference. Sarah, despite her anxiety and the pressure, managed to stabilise her patient, effectively preparing the ground for the surgeons. She stresses the need for ongoing training, which has given her the confidence to act quickly and effectively.

2. Benjamin: The challenge of pain
Benjamin talks about the times when he feels powerless in the face of his patients' intense pain. Despite painkillers and attentive care, the pain sometimes remains insurmountable. Yet it is at these difficult moments that he has learned to offer something else: a reassuring presence, a hand to hold, an attentive ear. Sometimes, the greatest victory is simply being there.

3. Leïla: Invisible victories

Leïla talks about the victories that are not always visible on the outside, but can be felt in the depths of the soul. She recalls a patient whose physical wounds were almost healed, but whose emotional scars were still raw. By working closely with psychologists and therapists, Leïla was able to help her patient find the strength to overcome her trauma.

4. Ahmed: The power of support

Ahmed emphasises the importance of teamwork in the burns unit. Each patient is a joint project, a shared mission. The nurses are not alone; they are supported by a team of dedicated professionals. Ahmed talks about the times when, exhausted, he drew strength from the support of his colleagues, turning challenges into shared victories.

5. Clémence: Restoring hope

For Clémence, the greatest victory is seeing a patient regain hope. She tells the story of a young man who, after a serious accident, had lost all will to live. Through dedicated care, constant encouragement and appropriate rehabilitation, she saw this patient gradually regain his zest for life, symbolising the reason she chose this profession.

These stories are just a few of many, but they offer a valuable insight into life in a burns unit. Every nurse, every health professional has their own challenges and triumphs, shaping the history of this very special medical field day by day.

Stories of resilience:
patients and their journeys

Resilience, the ability to bounce back in the face of adversity, is often at the heart of the lives of patients on the burns unit. Burns, whether accidental or intentional, have a profound effect not only on the body, but also on the mind. Yet, with the right support and unfailing determination, many patients manage to overcome their ordeals and reinvent themselves. Through some poignant stories, we discover the courage and perseverance of these broken, but never defeated, souls.

1. Amélie: Renaissance after the accident

Amélie was on holiday with her family when a badly controlled barbecue turned tragic. Burnt over 40% of her body, she had to cope not only with the physical pain, but also with readjusting to a new self-image. Thanks to a caring medical team and a close-knit family, Amélie has now got on with her life, bearing her scars like the scars of a warrior.

2. David: From street to renaissance

David was homeless when he was the victim of an attack that left him badly burnt. With no family to support him, the team at the burns unit became his new family. In addition to his physical care, he received psychosocial support to help him regain his self-confidence. Today, David is an active campaigner for the rights of the homeless and often talks about his resilience to inspire others.

3. Fatima: War scars and the quest for identity

Originally from a conflict zone, Fatima was the victim of a bombing raid. Evacuated and taken into care, she not only had to recover from her physical injuries but also overcome the trauma of war. Her care was complemented by intense psychological support, and thanks to the solidarity of numerous associations, she was able to start a new life in a country at peace.

4. Julien: The quest for forgiveness
Julien was burned in a laboratory accident when he was a chemistry student. Feeling guilty about his own injuries, he had to learn to forgive himself. His road to recovery was as much emotional as it was physical, and he stresses the crucial role of psychotherapy in his rehabilitation. Now a teacher, he teaches with passion, using his story as a lesson in resilience for his students.

5. Léa: Support as a pillar
Léa was still a baby when she was the victim of a house fire. Her devastated parents had to accompany her on her road to recovery. Her mother recounts their shared journey, recalling the challenges and the tears, but also the victories and the smiles. Léa is now a fulfilled teenager, and her family is living proof that with love and support, anything is possible.

These unique and inspiring stories are a reminder that resilience is a strength that lies dormant in all of us. It just needs to be awakened by hope, support and unshakeable determination.

Lessons learned from difficult situations

The journey of a nurse in a burns unit is paved with challenges. Each patient has a unique story, their own pain, and an internal battle to fight. But it is also in the midst of these moments of adversity that healthcare professionals draw invaluable lessons that forge their expertise and their humanity. By immersing ourselves in the most difficult situations, here are some of the timeless lessons that have been learned.

1. Active listening is therapeutic

Patients who have suffered severe burns do not only suffer from their physical injuries. The emotional and psychological pain is just as acute. Listening attentively, without judgement, can offer real solace, allowing patients to verbalise their fears, hopes and frustrations.

2. The importance of patience

Healing after a serious burn is a long and arduous process. Nurses must learn to manage their impatience and pass on this ability to wait to their patients. Every small improvement must be celebrated, while understanding that the road ahead will be long.

3. Flexibility is essential

Every burn and every patient is unique. What works for one may not work for another. Nurses must be prepared to adapt, to improvise and to find creative solutions to unexpected challenges.

4. Interdisciplinary collaboration is the key

Treating burn victims requires a holistic approach. From surgery to physiotherapy and psychological support, all professionals play a crucial role. Learning to work as a team, respecting each other's expertise and communicating effectively are key lessons.

5. Preservation for better care

Faced with daily pain and suffering, nurses can feel overwhelmed. They quickly learn the importance of taking care of themselves, recognising the signs of burnout and seeking support when necessary.

6. Celebrate every victory, no matter how small

In the often tense environment of a burns unit, it's essential to hold on to the positive moments. Every healing, every smile, every step towards recovery is a victory to celebrate.

7. Humanity first

Beyond the techniques, drugs and procedures, what remains engraved in the mind of the nurse is humanity. Compassion, empathy and respect are the pillars of care.

In the end, every difficult situation is an opportunity to learn and grow. These lessons, sometimes hard-won, are the foundation on which the excellence of the burns service rests.

Chapter 15:
THE NURSE,
PILLAR OF A MULTIDISCIPLINARY TEAM

Working with plastic surgeons

The field of plastic surgery is closely linked to that of burns. Reconstruction, grafting and aesthetic enhancement operations often call on the expertise of plastic surgeons. This is why collaboration between burns nurses and these surgeons is not only necessary, but essential. In this interdisciplinary environment, here's how the partnership between these two professionals manifests itself.

1. Pre-operative preparation
Before any surgical procedure, the nurse plays a vital role in preparing the patient. This involves assessing the patient's general condition, checking medical history, preparing the skin around the burn area and fitting the necessary medical devices. Collaboration with the plastic surgeon is essential to ensure that all conditions are optimal for surgery.

2. Support during the operation
Although the plastic surgeon is at the centre of the surgical act, the nurse remains an essential link in the process. He or she assists the surgeon, providing the necessary instruments, monitoring the patient's vital signs and ensuring that everything is carried out in optimal hygienic conditions.

3. Post-operative care
Once the operation is over, the nurse is often responsible for post-operative care. This care includes monitoring vital

signs, pain management, wound care, follow-up of grafts and prevention of complications. Regular communication with the plastic surgeon allows care to be adjusted as the patient progresses.

4. Education and advice
Nurses, with the support of plastic surgeons, play a vital role in patient education. They inform them about the stages to come, the precautions to take, the healing process, and answer their questions. This stage is crucial in reassuring patients and preparing them for the rest of their treatment.

5. Case reviews and discussions
The complexity of burns cases often requires interdisciplinary reviews. Nurses and plastic surgeons meet regularly to discuss cases, share observations and adjust treatment plans.

6. Further training
Plastic surgery is a constantly evolving field. As a result, nurses often have to undergo training to keep abreast of the latest techniques and discoveries. Plastic surgeons can play an essential role in sharing their knowledge and training teams.

In short, the relationship between the burns nurse and the plastic surgeon is symbiotic. Each brings his or her skills, know-how and passion to the healing of patients. Together, they form a solid team, capable of overcoming the most complex challenges.

Working with physiotherapists and occupational therapists

When a patient suffers serious burns, recovery is often a multidisciplinary process, with each professional making their own contribution. Among these professionals, physiotherapists and occupational therapists play a fundamental role, working hand in hand with nurses to ensure the physical and functional rehabilitation of patients.

1. Initial care and assessment
As soon as the patient is admitted, the nurse works closely with the physiotherapist to assess the extent and severity of the burns, as well as the potential impact on mobility. The occupational therapist assesses the patient's functional abilities, particularly with regard to activities of daily living.

2. Preventing after-effects
As burns heal, they can lead to contractures and stiff joints. The physiotherapist intervenes to ensure optimum mobility of the affected joints, while the nurse ensures that the skin is properly hydrated and elastic using topical treatments.

3. Functional rehabilitation
The occupational therapist is responsible for teaching the patient to carry out everyday tasks again, such as dressing, eating and writing. This collaboration is essential if patients are to regain their independence and live better with the after-effects of their injury.

4. Fitting orthoses
For some patients, orthoses may be necessary to prevent or treat deformities. The occupational therapist, in collaboration with the nurse, determines the need, type and timing of these devices.

5. Pain management
The physiotherapist often provides non-medicinal solutions for pain management, such as specific exercises or relaxation techniques. The nurse, for his part, can adjust the drug treatment according to the feedback from the physiotherapist and the patient's needs.

6. Long-term follow-up
Even after discharge from hospital, the collaboration does not stop. Nurses, physiotherapists and occupational therapists often work together to provide follow-up care at home, to ensure that the patient continues to progress and to adapt care as the situation evolves.

7. Education and advice
The three professionals play a crucial role in patient education. They offer practical advice, techniques for better day-to-day living and resources to help them better understand and manage their injuries.

The collaboration between the nurse, the physiotherapist and the occupational therapist is a precious alliance that aims for the optimal well-being of the patient. Each professional brings his or her own speciality, but it is together, through their joint work, that they enable the patient to return to as normal a life as possible after a trauma as severe as a major burn.

The importance of communication with the family

Communication with the family is at the heart of care for burn patients. These often traumatic injuries leave not only physical scars, but also emotional ones, both for the patient and for their loved ones. As a nurse in a burns unit, the ability to establish a relationship of trust with the family is as essential as the direct care given to the patient.

1. Reassurance in critical moments
When a patient with severe burns is admitted to hospital, the family is often overwhelmed by fear and anxiety. The first few hours are crucial for establishing a dialogue. The nurse must provide clear information about the patient's condition, forthcoming procedures and prognosis. This transparency helps to reassure the family and **prepare** them for **the challenges ahead.**

2. Sharing progress and challenges
Healing burns is a long process, often fraught with complications. Keeping the family regularly informed of progress, but also of obstacles, is essential to maintaining a relationship of trust. This allows the family to understand the care pathway, prepare themselves mentally and adjust their support accordingly.

3. Emotional and psychological support
The role of the nurse is not limited to medical communication. Listening to the concerns, fears and doubts of loved ones is essential. Referring them to professionals, such as psychologists or support groups, can be beneficial in helping them manage the stress and emotional shock.

4. Training and education
As the patient gets closer to discharge, the nurse plays a crucial role in educating the family. This involves training them in home care, in recognising the signs of complications and in the patient's specific needs in terms of nutrition, hygiene and exercise.

5. Facilitating family involvement

Encouraging the family to take an active part in care can improve the patient's experience. Whether it's helping with mobilisation, taking part in physiotherapy sessions or simply being present during day-to-day care, their involvement is a source of encouragement and comfort for the patient.

6. Respect family dynamics

Every family is unique. Nurses must respect cultural, religious and individual differences, while ensuring that the patient's needs remain paramount.

Communication with the family is not just a professional obligation, but a human necessity. By cultivating a solid relationship with their loved ones, nurses facilitate the patient's recovery, while offering essential support to those around them. This two-way communication is the cornerstone of holistic care, where emotional and psychological well-being are just as important as physical health.

Chapter 16:
CAREER DEVELOPMENT
IN BURN CARE

Training and specialisation

In today's ever-changing medical world, continuing education and specialisation have become the norm for healthcare professionals, particularly those working in fields as demanding and specific as burns care. For nurses, this is essential not only to provide the best possible care, but also to progress in their careers.

1. Initial training
All nurses begin with initial training that covers the basics of nursing care. However, to work in a specialised unit such as a burns unit, additional training, generally provided by the hospital or an affiliated institution, is required to familiarise them with the procedures and techniques specific to this field.

2. Specialisation
Post-graduate training programmes are available for those wishing to specialise in burn care. These programmes cover advanced care techniques, the pathophysiology of burns, pain management and communication with patients and their families.

3. Ongoing training
Medicine and care techniques are evolving rapidly. To stay up to date, nurses need to engage in continuing education. Whether through workshops, webinars, conferences or courses, these learning opportunities are essential to maintaining and improving the quality of care.

4. Research and publications

Taking part in clinical studies or writing articles for specialist journals can enable nurses to expand their knowledge, while contributing to the advancement of the discipline.

5. Professional certifications

Obtaining certification in specific areas, such as pain management or reconstructive surgery, can not only raise a nurse's level of competence, but also strengthen their professional credibility.

6. Professional networks

Joining professional associations or specialty groups can offer countless benefits, from networking and access to educational resources to defending the rights and interests of specialist nurses.

Training and specialisation is an ongoing process that requires dedication, passion and commitment. For nurses, it's a never-ending quest for excellence that guarantees not only better quality care for patients, but also a rewarding and fulfilling career. The key is to remain curious, open to innovation and always ready to learn.

Managing stress and preventing burnout

The nursing profession, especially in specialised units such as the burn unit, is stressful by nature. Faced with often dramatic situations, nurses must remain professional, caring and efficient, while managing their own emotions. It is therefore crucial to recognise the signs of stress, understand the causes and put in place strategies to prevent burnout.

1. Understanding the origins of stress

Stress can have several causes:

- **Emotional demands**: Watching patients suffer on a daily basis, sometimes with no hope of rapid improvement, is emotionally taxing.
- **Workload**: The large number of patients, administrative tasks and irregular working hours can be a source of stress.
- **Complex care**: Burn patients require complex care and constant monitoring.
- **Interactions**: Communication with patients' families, surgeons or other medical staff can be a source of tension.

2. Recognising the warning signs of burnout

Burnout does not happen overnight. Warning signs such as persistent fatigue, irritability, reduced job satisfaction, sleep disturbances and depressive symptoms should raise the alarm.

3. Setting up adaptation mechanisms

- **Work/life balance**: It's essential to draw a clear line between work time and personal time to recharge your batteries.
- **Regular breaks**: Short breaks during the day help you to relax and reduce tension.
- **Social support**: Talking to colleagues, friends or family members can help relieve stress.

4. Professional strategies

- **Supervision and mentoring**: Having a mentor or supervisor with whom to discuss difficult cases can be very beneficial.
- **Ongoing training**: Training can offer new techniques or perspectives for managing stressful situations.

5. Taking care of yourself
- **Physical activity**: Helps reduce stress and improve mental health.
- **Meditation and relaxation**: These techniques help to manage stress and anxiety.
- **Professional consultation**: Psychologists or therapists can offer tailored strategies for managing stress.

Stress management and burnout prevention are not luxuries, but a necessity for every healthcare professional. Taking care of yourself also means being able to take care of others in the best possible way. So it's essential to listen to yourself and your emotions, and not hesitate to seek help when you need it.

Taking part in research and innovation

The medical world is constantly evolving, driven by unprecedented technological and scientific advances. For burns nurses, getting involved in research and innovation is not only an opportunity for professional enrichment, but also a chance to improve the quality of care offered to patients. Here's how a nurse can play an active part in the dynamics of research and innovation.

1. Understanding the importance of nursing research
- **Benefits for patients**: The aim of the research is to improve care methods, resulting in better patient care.
- **Contribution to the profession**: Participating in research enriches the nursing field, enhances the role of carers and strengthens their position in the multidisciplinary medical team.

2. Training in research methodology
- **Workshops and training**: Many institutions offer training in research methods, article writing and research ethics.
- **Interdisciplinary collaboration**: Working alongside researchers from other specialities can offer an enriching perspective and broaden nurses' skills.

3. Participate in clinical trials
- **Patient recruitment**: The nurse's proximity to patients can play a key role in their inclusion in clinical trials.
- **Data collection**: Nurses are often involved in data collection and analysis, thanks to their in-depth knowledge of the patient pathway.

4. Working with the medical industries
- **Evaluation of new equipment**: Medical equipment manufacturers regularly ask carers to test and evaluate new devices.
- **Attending trade fairs and conferences**: This is an opportunity for nurses to discover the latest innovations, but also to share their expertise with industry professionals.

5. Contribute to publications
- **Writing articles**: Sharing your experiences, studies and thoughts in specialist journals helps to advance knowledge in the field.
- **Critical reading**: Nurses may also be asked to assess the quality and relevance of articles submitted to professional journals.

6. Encourage a culture of innovation within the team
- **Discussions and brainstorming**: team meetings are a great opportunity to share innovative ideas and feedback.
- **Scientific watch**: Keeping an eye on the latest publications, studies and conferences helps you stay up to date and incorporate best practice quickly.

Nurses, by virtue of their central position in patient care, have a unique vision of the needs and challenges of care. This perspective is crucial to research and innovation. By playing an active role, nurses help to develop practices for the benefit of patients, the profession and the medical community as a whole.

Chapter 17:
CONCLUSION: THE NURSE, GUARDIAN OF HOPE AND HEALING

The department's successes and challenges

Working in the burns unit is an exercise that constantly oscillates between moments of great satisfaction and often formidable challenges. It's a place where human life is constantly in the balance, where every gesture counts and every decision can have lasting consequences. Let's immerse ourselves in this world of contrasts, to discover the successes that inspire and the challenges that motivate us to constantly improve.

Success stories: Testimonies of a resilient force
1. Spectacular rescues:
There are these cases, these stories of patients who arrived with very poor prognoses, but who, thanks to the team's expertise, have not only survived but have also regained a quality of life. These success stories are living reminders of the impact of the work carried out in the department.

2. Innovation and adoption of new techniques:
The adoption of new methods, whether skin grafts, dressing techniques or therapies, demonstrates the department's ability to evolve and incorporate best practice to improve care.

3. Team cohesion:
Faced with often trying situations, the unity of the team is an achievement in itself. This professional solidarity is crucial to overcoming difficulties.

4. Professional recognition:
The contribution of the burns unit is regularly recognised at conferences, training courses and in specialist publications, highlighting the quality of the care and research carried out.

The challenges: Seeking better care
1. Pain management:
Pain is a constant companion for patients with severe burns. Despite progress, pain management remains a challenge, balancing effective relief with the side effects of medication.

2. Infection prevention:
Infections are a constant threat to burn patients, due to the broken skin barrier. Ensuring a sterile environment and rapidly treating any infection is a daily battle.

3. Psychological support:
In addition to physical care, psychological care for patients and their families is essential, given the trauma of burns and the challenges of rehabilitation.

4. Limited resources:
As in many specialist services, resources - whether human, material or financial - are often stretched, requiring constant optimisation.

5. Continuing education:
The world of medicine is changing fast, and keeping up to date with the latest techniques, research and innovations is a challenge in itself.

Every day, the burns unit experiences successes that reinforce the conviction in the mission accomplished, but it is also confronted with challenges that push it to go ever further in the excellence of its care. This duality, between celebrating victories and confronting obstacles, is the reflection of a profession dedicated to life, in all its complexity and beauty.

Inspiring testimonials
nurses and patients

Marie, a nurse for 10 years in the burns unit:
"When I joined this department, I didn't really know what to expect. I was surprised by the complexity and rigour involved in caring for burn patients. But what struck me most were the intense moments of humanity. I saw patients who, despite unbearable pain, showed incredible resilience. I saw families come together with strength and hope. And through all this, I've learnt the true essence of my profession: not only to treat, but also to accompany, support and witness these little everyday miracles."

Lucas, victim of a gas explosion, patient :
"After the accident, I no longer recognised my reflection in the mirror. Physically and mentally, I was shattered. But as soon as I arrived at the hospital, I was surrounded by a dedicated and caring team. The nurses were my pillars, my guides through this ordeal. Their empathy, patience and skill made all the difference. Today, I wear my scars like badges of honour, reminders of this battle I fought with the help of an exceptional team."

Julien, nurse specialising in reconstructive surgery:
"Every day, we face immense challenges. But what motivates me is to see these patients, who have lost

everything, gradually coming back to life. Helping them to regain their self-esteem and self-confidence takes time, listening and a lot of love. And when they come back, months or years later, to show us their progress, their new life, I tell myself that all the effort has been worthwhile".

Sophie, burned in a domestic accident, is patient:
"I was angry at myself, at the world. Why was I angry at myself? But thanks to the medical team, I learned to transform that anger into positive energy. The nurses taught me to embrace my new image, to see it as a strength rather than a weakness. They were much more than just carers. They were my therapists, my confidants, my friends."

Léa, intensive care nurse :
"The hardest days are those when, despite all our efforts, we can't save a patient. On those days, the weight of our responsibility weighs heavily on us. But what keeps me going is thinking about all the people we've helped, all the lives we've touched. And I realise that every smile, every thank you, every tear shed is proof that our work has deep meaning."

These testimonials reflect the harsh reality, but also the beauty and strength, of the burns service. They illustrate the deep interconnection between carers and patients, and serve as a reminder of the crucial importance of empathy, expertise and determination in the healing journey.

A vision for the future:
Innovation and continuous improvement

The world of medicine is constantly evolving, with each decade bringing new discoveries, techniques and innovations. The field of burns is no exception. The management of burn patients, once focused primarily on survival, has gradually broadened to encompass a more global vision of rehabilitation, well-being and quality of life.

Cutting-edge technologies :
Technological advances are revolutionising the way burns are treated. 3D printers, for example, now make it possible to create personalised skin grafts, optimising healing and reducing the risk of rejection. Intelligent dressings, capable of releasing drugs in a controlled manner or monitoring the state of the wound in real time, are also at the forefront of the transformation of care.

Holistic approach :
The future also holds the promise of a more holistic approach to care. Recognising that burns affect not only the body but also the mind, initiatives integrating psychology, physiotherapy, art therapy and other forms of complementary care are multiplying to offer holistic healing.

Research and international collaboration :
International collaboration is intensifying, and healthcare professionals are increasingly sharing their techniques, discoveries and best practices. These exchanges lead to continuous improvement in the care offered to patients. The major world congresses on burns bear witness to this desire to pool skills and move forward together.

Continuing education :
To stay at the cutting edge, nurses and all care staff need to be constantly learning. Ongoing training programmes, simulations and specialised courses are all ways of ensuring that every patient benefits from the best techniques and approaches available.

Listening to the patient :
Increasingly, medicine is moving towards listening more closely to the patient. Patients, who used to be passive, are now becoming active players in their own healing, with their feelings, needs and suggestions being integrated into the treatment process.

So the future of the burns service is full of promise. With a combination of technological innovation, a holistic approach and borderless collaboration, the future looks bright for offering burn patients a new chance, a life full of possibilities and hope.

www.ingramcontent.com/pod-product-compliance
Lightning Source LLC
Chambersburg PA
CBHW062328290526
45794CB00005B/1940